In Clinical Practice

T0281284

More information about this series at http://www.springer.com/series/13483

Abdul Qayyum Rana
Kelvin L. Chou

Essential Tremor
in Clinical Practice

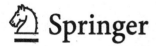 Springer

Abdul Qayyum Rana
Parkinson's Clinic of Eastern
    Toronto & Movement
    Disorders Centre
Toronto, ON, Canada

Kelvin L. Chou
Michigan House
University of Michigan
    Medical School
Ann Arbor, MI, USA

ISSN 2199-6652   ISSN 2199-6660   (electronic)
In Clinical Practice
ISBN 978-3-319-14597-6   ISBN 978-3-319-14598-3   (eBook)
DOI 10.1007/978-3-319-14598-3

Library of Congress Control Number: 2015932231

Springer Cham Heidelberg New York Dordrecht London
© Springer International Publishing Switzerland 2015
This work is subject to copyright. All rights are reserved by the Publisher, whether the whole or part of the material is concerned, specifically the rights of translation, reprinting, reuse of illustrations, recitation, broadcasting, reproduction on microfilms or in any other physical way, and transmission or information storage and retrieval, electronic adaptation, computer software, or by similar or dissimilar methodology now known or hereafter developed.
The use of general descriptive names, registered names, trademarks, service marks, etc. in this publication does not imply, even in the absence of a specific statement, that such names are exempt from the relevant protective laws and regulations and therefore free for general use.
The publisher, the authors and the editors are safe to assume that the advice and information in this book are believed to be true and accurate at the date of publication. Neither the publisher nor the authors or the editors give a warranty, express or implied, with respect to the material contained herein or for any errors or omissions that may have been made.

Printed on acid-free paper

Springer International Publishing AG Switzerland is part of Springer Science+Business Media (www.springer.com)

Preface

"Essential Tremor" is the most common movement disorder, which may be mild in severity, and therefore may not come to medical attention in many cases. However, essential tremor is sometimes quite debilitating and may interfere with one's daily activities. Though there is no cure for essential tremor, the last decade has brought about many new advances in treatment for this condition, including deep brain stimulation, MRI-guided focused ultrasound, and even non-invasive treatments such as the Liftware spoon. Because essential tremor is often thought of as "benign", many medical professionals may not be aware of these cutting edge, newer treatments.

This guide concisely covers the phenomenology, etiology, pathophysiology, symptoms and different treatments available for this condition. This book is geared towards medical professionals that see patients with essential tremor, including internists, general and family practitioners, geriatricians, neurologists, fellows and residents in training in neurology, internal medicine and family practice, nurse practitioners and physician assistants in neurology clinics, nurses, physical/occupational therapists, and medical students. Every effort has been made to present correct and up-to-date information in this handbook, but medicine is a field with ongoing research and developments.

We are grateful to Ashfique Adlul, Ryhana Dawood and Mohammad Abdullah Rana for proofreading, as well as other students who assisted during this project. We are thankful to Dr. Paul Jensen, Dr. Tilak Mendis, Dr. Emmanuelle Pourcher, and Dr. Frederic Calon, who reviewed this publication and provided very useful suggestions on various sections. We are especially thankful to Dr. Afshan Rana for her input as an internist especially about the section on medical treatments of essential tremor.

We are grateful to Evelyn Shifflett, who drew all of the illustrations in this book, except for two. We would like to thank Chris Winters for the illustration on the deep brain stimulation system, and John Redmond for the illustration depicting the Liftware spoon. Suggestions to improve this book are welcome and should be forwarded to the authors directly.

Toronto, ON, Canada   Abdul Qayyum Rana
Ann Arbor, MI, USA   Kelvin L. Chou

Contents

Chapter 1
What Is Tremor?

Definition of Tremor

Tremor is defined as an involuntary rhythmic oscillation of a body part, mediated by alternating contractions of reciprocally acting muscles [1]. Patients who complain of shaking or tremulousness may not always have tremor. Its rhythmicity often allows it to be differentiated from other involuntary movements such as myoclonus, clonus, chorea, dystonia, and tics [2]. Essential tremor is the most common tremor disorder, as well as the most common movement disorder (see Chap. 3 for how to diagnose essential tremor) [3].

Classification of Tremor

Tremor can be classified in a number of ways [4, 5]:

(A) According to position of the body part affected by tremor
   Tremor can be categorized as a resting tremor (if the tremor occurs while the affected body part is in complete repose) or an action tremor (if there is voluntary muscle activity in the affected body part) [4]. Action tremor can be further subdivided into postural tremor or kinetic tremor (see "Terminology of Tremor" below) [6].

A.Q. Rana, K.L. Chou, *Essential Tremor in Clinical Practice*,
In Clinical Practice, DOI 10.1007/978-3-319-14598-3_1,
© Springer International Publishing Switzerland 2015

(B) According to the regions of body affected

Tremor may affect different body parts including limbs, head, tongue, jaw, vocal cords and palate. The parts of the body that are affected by tremor depend upon the underlying neurological condition. As an example, essential tremor commonly affects the hands, head and voice while Parkinson disease patients may have tremors in the arms, legs, and chin, but rarely the head [7, 8].

(C) According to the frequency of tremor (Table 1.1)

1. Low frequency tremor (3–6 Hz) e.g. tremor of Parkinson disease [9]
2. Medium frequency tremor (7–14 Hz) e.g. ET or enhanced physiologic tremor [10]
3. High frequency tremor e.g. (>14 Hz) e.g. Orthostatic tremor [4]

It should be noted that there is great overlap in tremor frequencies between disorders. Essential tremor patients,

TABLE 1.1 Frequencies of different tremor syndromes [5]

Tremor syndrome	Frequency HZ
Enhanced physiological tremor	10–14
Essential tremor syndrome	4–12
Primary orthostatic tremor	14–18
Task specific tremor	4–8
Holmes tremor	3–5
Tremor of Parkinson disease	3–7
Cerebellar tremor	3–5
Palatal tremor	2–6
Dystonic tremor	5–7
Alcoholic tremor	3–4
Toxic and drug induced tremor	5–10
Psychogenic tremor	Variable

especially those who have large amplitude tremors, may have tremor frequencies in the 3–6 Hz range, while Parkinson disease patients may have tremors with a frequency >6 Hz [9, 10].

(D) According to the amplitude of tremor

1. Mild amplitude (<2 cm)
2. Moderate amplitude (2–4 cm)
3. Severe amplitude (>4 cm)

(E) According to the etiology of tremor

1. Essential tremor
2. Enhanced physiological tremor
3. Drug or toxin induced tremor.
4. Dystonic tremor
5. Cerebellar tremor
6. Holmes tremor (mid brain tremor)
7. Primary orthostatic tremor.
8. Cortical tremor
9. Neuropathy associated tremor.
10. Tremor of Parkinson disease.
11. Psychogenic tremor
12. Tremor is also seen in many other medical conditions such as thyroid disease, Wilson disease, hypoxia, hypotension, AIDS, hereditary hemochromatosis.
13. Task specific tremor such as primary writing tremor.
14. Post traumatic tremor

Terminology of Tremor

Resting Tremor

Resting tremor is evident when the affected body part is in complete repose, supported against gravity and is not voluntarily activated [2, 4]. During the onset of voluntary activity, the tremor completely disappears or the amplitude of the tremor becomes less prominent.

The presence of a pure rest tremor suggests parkinsonism [6]. There may be many causes of parkinsonism, including:

(A) Parkinson disease
(B) Atypical parkinsonism (Multiple system atrophy, Dementia with Lewy bodies, Progressive Supranuclear Palsy)
(C) Drug-induced parkinsonism

Action Tremor

Action tremor occurs during voluntary activity of the affected body part or when the affected body part is maintaining a steady posture against gravity, and diminishes or completely disappears at rest [2, 4]. There are four subtypes of action tremor [6].

(A) Postural tremor
   This subtype of action tremor occurs when the affected body part is maintaining a posture against gravity [4, 6].
(B) Kinetic tremor
   This subtype of action tremor occurs when the affected body part is performing a voluntary activity which could be goal directed or non goal directed [4, 6]. An *intention tremor* is a subtype of kinetic tremor, where the amplitude of the tremor increases when the affected body part is approaching a target [4, 6]. The use of the term intention tremor typically implies cerebellar pathology.
(C) Isometric tremor
   This subtype occurs when the affected body part performs muscle contractions without movement (such as fist-clenching or standing) [4, 6].
(D) Task-specific tremor
   This type of tremor occurs during a specific activity such as only when writing [4, 6].

Conditions that may cause a primary action tremor include [5]:

(a) Enhanced physiological tremor
(b) Anxiety or emotional stress.
(c) Metabolic: hypoglycemia, thyrotoxicosis, pheochromo-cytoma, adrenocorticosteroids
(d) Drugs and toxins: beta agonists, amphetamines, theo-phylline, caffeine and alcohol withdrawal, etc.
(e) Essential tremor
(f) Primary writing tremor
(g) Orthostatic tremor
(h) Cerebellar tremor
(i) Neuropathic tremor
(j) Dystonic tremor

Mixed Rest/Action Tremor

Some diagnoses can present with either a rest or an action tremor [5]:

(a) Drug-induced
(b) Wilson disease
(c) Psychogenic

Other diagnoses may have equal rest and action compo-nents to the tremor [5]:

(a) Drug-induced tremor
(b) Wilson disease
(c) Psychogenic tremor
(d) Holmes tremor
(e) Parkinson disease when tremor is severe
(f) Essential tremor when severe may have a resting compo-nent if limbs not fully relaxed

Description of Tremor

When approaching a patient who presents with tremor, it should be first categorized according to its positional properties (rest or action tremor) [6]. While this is often straightforward, some patients may have both rest and action tremors (see Mixed Rest/Action Tremors). When this happens, other classifications may help in coming up with a differential.

The following parameters should be included when describing a particular tremor:

1. The position of affected body part in which tremor is most prominent (eg: rest, postural, activity, specific task)
2. Topography (eg: head, limbs, chin, jaw, etc.)
3. The frequency of the tremor
4. The amplitude of tremor

References

1. Zesiewicz TA, Hauser RA. Phenomenology and treatment of tremor disorders. Neurol Clin. 2001;19:651–80.
2. Elias WJ, Shah BB. Tremor. JAMA. 2014;311:948–54.
3. Louis ED, Ottman R, Hauser WA. How common is the most common adult movement disorder? Estimates of the prevalence of essential tremor throughout the world. Mov Disord. 1998;13:5–10.
4. Deuschl G, Bain P, Brin M. Consensus statement of the Movement Disorder Society on Tremor. Ad Hoc Scientific Committee. Mov Disord. 1998;13 Suppl 3:2–23.
5. Fahn S, Jankovic J. Tremors: diagnosis and treatment. In: Fahn S, Jankovic J, editors. Principles and practice of movement disorders. Philadelphia: Churchill Livingstone Elsevier; 2007. p. 451–78.
6. Chou KL. Diagnosis and management of the patient with tremor. Med Health R I. 2004;87:135–8.
7. Samii A. Cardinal features of early Parkinson's disease. In: Factor SA, Weiner WJ, editors. Parkinson's disease: diagnosis and clinical management. 2nd ed. New York: Demos Medical Publishing, Inc.; 2008. p. 41–56.

8. Jankovic J. Essential tremor: clinical characteristics. Neurology. 2000;54:S21–5.
9. Findley LJ, Gresty MA, Halmagyi GM. Tremor, the cogwheel phenomenon and clonus in Parkinson's disease. J Neurol Neurosurg Psychiatry. 1981;44:534–46.
10. Elble RJ, Higgins C, Leffler K, Hughes L. Factors influencing the amplitude and frequency of essential tremor. Mov Disord. 1994;9:589–96.

Chapter 2
What Is Essential Tremor?

Essential tremor (ET) is one of the most common neurological disorders and is characterized by the presence of action tremor of the hands [1]. It is also known variably in the medical literature as Familial Essential Tremor and Benign Essential Tremor. The use of "benign" in front of ET is misleading, as the tremor may be quite disabling [2, 3]. Similarly, not all cases of ET are familial. Thus, the condition is best termed "Essential Tremor".

Epidemiology

ET can affect anyone at any age. Based on tertiary center referrals, the distribution of age at onset is bimodal, with a small peak at around 20 years of age and another one around 60 years of age [4–6], though in population based studies, there may be just one large peak later in life [6]. About 5–15 % of ET cases occur during childhood [4, 6, 7]. Prevalence estimates vary widely because of differing diagnostic criteria, but is present in approximately 1 % of the general population, approximately 4–5.6 % of patients aged 40 or older [8, 9], and approximately 6–9 % of patients aged 60 or older [1, 8, 9]. An age-associated increase in the prevalence of ET is consistently found across all studies [1, 9]. Applying these prevalence rates to United States census figures, almost five million people in the United States

A.Q. Rana, K.L. Chou, *Essential Tremor in Clinical Practice*,
In Clinical Practice, DOI 10.1007/978-3-319-14598-3_2,
© Springer International Publishing Switzerland 2015

over the age of 40 are affected with ET. Overall, tremor appears to occur with similar frequency in men and women [4]. This condition is common in all races across the world, though may be slightly higher in Caucasians than African-Americans [10].

Genetics/Environmental Risk Factors

The exact cause of ET is unknown. Because patients with ET are five times more likely to have first degree relatives with tremor compared to the general population, it is largely considered a genetic disorder [11]. The genetics of ET, however, are not yet clear. In a significant number of cases, ET is hereditary and transmitted in an autosomal dominant pattern. Mutations in chromosome 2p22-25, 3q13, 6p23, and the fused in sarcoma (FUS) gene have been suggested to be the disease loci in some of these dominantly inherited families, though there are families with dominantly inherited ET without a link to these loci [12–16]. Genome-wide association studies have identified sequence variations in the LINGO1 (leucine-rich repeat and Ig domain containing 1) and SLC1A2 (glial glutamate transporter) genes in European subjects as possible genetic risk factors for ET [16].

Up to 50 % of ET patients do not have affected relatives, suggesting that environmental factors may also play a role [17]. This is supported by the lack of complete concordance in monozygotic twins with ET [18] and the existence of wide differences in age of onset and severity of tremor within families. Harmane (1-methyl-9H-pyrido[3,4-b]indole) has turned out to be an intriguing possible environmental toxin connected to ET. Harmane is a tremor-producing β-carboline alkaloid found in cooked meat, and elevated blood and brain harmane concentrations have been found in ET patients in large case-control studies [18–20]. There have also been associations between lead and pesticide exposure and ET, but more work is needed to more firmly establish all of these toxins as definitive risk factors [18].

Pathophysiology

The pathophysiological mechanisms of ET are poorly under-stood. Central nervous system pathology is supported by the observation that thalamotomy, thalamic deep brain stimula-tion and centrally acting drugs may improve tremor [21, 22]. The cerebellum in particular may play an important role in pathophysiology of ET. It has been suggested that ET origi-nates from the inferior olivary nucleus of the cerebellum, in cells displaying inherent oscillatory-pacemaking properties [23]. These central oscillators are normally kept in check by inhibitors such as the neurotransmitter GABA, but such a mechanism could be defective in ET [24]. Abnormal oscilla-tion would then propagate through the cerebello-thalamo-cortical network, resulting in tremors. This theory is supported by findings that lesions or injury of regions within the thala-mus where the cerebellum sends its information reduces the intensity of ET [22, 25, 26]. Neuronal discharges correlated with tremor have been observed to occur in the ventrolateral thalamus, particularly in the ventralis intermedius nucleus [27]. Contralateral limb tremor can be suppressed by the ablation or high frequency stimulation of the ventralis inter-medius nucleus of thalamus [22, 28].

The neuropathology of ET is controversial. There have been some studies reporting neurodegenerative changes in the cerebellum of patients with ET, including Purkinje cell loss, increased Purkinje cell axon swelling (torpedos), and decreased Purkinje cell linear density [29, 30]. However, other clinicopathologic studies of ET have reported no sig-nificant cerebellar pathology [31, 32]. Thus it remains unclear if ET is a neurodegenerative disorder.

Clinical Presentation

Tremor Characteristics

The hallmark of ET is an action (kinetic and postural) tremor of the hands [4, 5]. This is different from the tremor seen in

Parkinson disease, which is a rest tremor (tremors improve with use of the affected limb) [33]. A variety of common tasks may be affected in ET. Writing may be tremulous, and the size of handwriting is usually large (macrographia). This in contrast to Parkinson disease, in which the size of handwriting typically becomes small (micrographia) [33]. When tremor is severe, patients may not be able to sign checks and may even have difficulty keeping the pen on the paper. ET patients also report trouble holding objects like a cup of coffee, and can have problems using utensils to eat. When moderate, they may spill liquids or food and many develop ways of accommodating the tremor, such as using two hands to hold a cup or by filling their cups partway. When in public, patients may avoid ordering certain menu items such as soup because of the potential for embarrassment [34]. In some cases, patients' tremors may be so severe that they need to put lids on their cups or drink from a straw in order not to spill. Other tasks that may be affected by the tremor in ET include dressing, shaking, putting on makeup, putting keys in locks, and using a screwdriver.

Tremor frequency in ET may range from 4 to 12 Hz, but is more typically in the range of 7–10 Hz [35, 36]. The tremor frequency usually slows down with age, at a rate of about 0.07 Hz per year [37]. This decrease in frequency causes a gradual increase in tremor amplitude over the years. In fact, ET patients with high amplitude tremors often oscillate at a lower frequency [38]. On examination, ET typically causes a flexion extension movement at the wrists, and/or abduction movement of the fingers. A pronation-supination (pill-rolling) tremor of the hands is more typical of Parkinson disease and is present in ET in only a minority of cases.

The tremor of ET is usually symmetric or only mildly asymmetric [4, 5]. The presence of unilateral hand tremor would be more consistent with the presence of other conditions, like early Parkinson disease, focal dystonia or primary writing tremor. Though ET and Parkinson disease are distinct clinical entities, there is some evidence that the 2 disorders may overlap. In some family studies of Parkinson disease, there is a co-occurrence of ET above what would be expected by chance alone [39, 40]. Additionally, some studies have reported an increased risk of developing Parkinson disease/Parkinsonism in ET patients [41, 42]. Other studies have indicated that the prevalence of preceding ET among a population of Parkinson disease patients is not higher than the prevalence of ET in the general population [43]. These conflicting findings may be due to varying definitions of ET and the different methods of ascertainment. Future studies will hopefully clarify the connection between ET and PD.

As mentioned earlier (see Genetics/Environmental Risk Factors), patients often have a family history of tremors. Most patients with ET seek attention only if they have a functional or social disability because of tremor. ET may result in social phobia due to embarrassment. Embarrassment is present in nearly half of ET cases with no head tremor and only mild arm tremor, so severity of tremor is not associated with embarrassment [34]. Younger patients and women tend to have more embarrassment, and the presence of embarrassment is associated with greater medication use [34].

Other Body Parts Affected

Though ET typically affects the upper extremities and the hands, it may also involve other body parts. Typically, the tremor spreads upwards to the head, then the voice [4, 5]. Tremor may also affect the legs, jaw, tongue, and trunk, though not as often as the head and voice [4, 5]. If these other body regions (head, voice, legs, jaw, tongue, and trunk) are involved, the tremors typically occur in conjunction with hand tremor and are rarely present in isolation [4, 5]. The presence of isolated head tremor suggests cervical dystonia, while an isolated voice tremor suggests laryngeal dystonia [44].

ET head tremor may be in a "no-no" or a "yes-yes" direction [4]. A rotatory head tremor suggests the possibility of cervical dystonia. Patients are often unaware of their head tremor and know they have it only because others point it out [45]. Women with essential tremor are more likely to develop a head tremor [44]. Voice tremor is generally of insidious onset. Patients may complain of voice changes and an increased effort to speak, but not necessarily a voice tremor. Women and patients with an older age of tremor onset are more likely to develop voice tremor [46]. Jaw tremor is typically associated with more severe and wide-spread tremor involvement [47]. Jaw tremor in ET may be confused with the perioral tremor of Parkinson disease, in which the lower lip and chin are affected.

Exacerbating/Alleviating Factors

Fatigue, stress, central nervous system stimulation, sexual arousal, emotional excitement and temperature extremes can exacerbate the tremor in ET [4]. In up to 60–70 % of ET patients, tremor is dampened by intake of alcohol [4, 5]. The effect of alcohol seems to be centrally mediated [21]. The history of response to alcohol is helpful diagnostically, though it does not have to be present to make the diagnosis. Caffeine on the other hand, may precipitate tremor. ET, like most other movement disorders, disappears in sleep. Occasionally, patients may complain of an especially coarse tremor upon awakening in the morning.

Other Associated Motor and Non-motor Features

It should be noted that studies on other features of ET are somewhat controversial and inconclusive. Gait abnormalities have been reported in patients with ET, including postural instability and ataxia [48, 49]. These gait changes are beyond that seen with normal aging, and may result from cerebellar dysfunction. Mild eye movement abnormalities have also been reported in ET patients [50]. Non-motor features that have been reported in ET include cognitive problems, personality changes, and depression/anxiety [2, 51]. Cognitive deficits are typically mild in nature, especially when compared to patients with Alzheimer's disease and Parkinson disease, and detectable only with sophisticated neuropsychological tests [2, 51–53]. Attention and executive function seem to be the cognitive domains that are consistently reported to be affected [53]. Several studies have reported that older onset of ET is associated with an increased risk of developing dementia [54, 55], but it is still not clear if this is due to ET or aging. A shy, doubtful and worrisome personality has also been associated with ET [56, 57], but another study instead found ET associated with more aggressiveness and hostility [58]. ET is associated with higher anxiety scores and higher levels of depression than in the general community [58, 59]. It is unclear if this is due to underlying pathophysiology of ET, the presence of tremor, embarrassment from tremor, or all of the above.

Disease Progression

ET typically worsens over time, though progression is not linear. As the amplitude of tremor increases, the frequency of tremor may decrease [37]. Of those ET patients who seek medical care, more than 90 % of them report disability from the tremors [60]. Up to a quarter of ET patients are forced into early retirement [2, 4]. In general, it has been reported that ET does not affect life expectancy, though there is a population-based study suggesting a 45 % increased risk of mortality in ET [61].

References

1. Louis ED, Ottman R, Hauser WA. How common is the most common adult movement disorder? Estimates of the prevalence of essential tremor throughout the world. Mov Disord. 1998;13:5–10.
2. Louis ED, Okun MS. It is time to remove the 'benign' from the essential tremor label. Parkinsonism Relat Disord. 2011;17:516–20.
3. Busenbark KL, Nash J, Nash S, Hubble JP, Koller WC. Is essential tremor benign? Neurology. 1991;41:1982–3.

4. Bain PG, Findley LJ, Thompson PD, et al. A study of hereditary essential tremor. Brain. 1994;117(Pt 4):805–24.
5. Lou JS, Jankovic J. Essential tremor: clinical correlates in 350 patients. Neurology. 1991;41:234–8.
6. Louis ED, Dogu O. Does age of onset in essential tremor have a bimodal distribution? Data from a tertiary referral setting and a population-based study. Neuroepidemiology. 2007;29:208–12.
7. Louis ED, Dure LS, Pullman S. Essential tremor in childhood: a series of nineteen cases. Mov Disord. 2001;16:921–3.
8. Rautakorpi I, Takala J, Marttila RJ, Sievers K, Rinne UK. Essential tremor in a Finnish population. Acta Neurol Scand. 1982;66:58–67.
9. Dogu O, Sevim S, Camdeviren H, et al. Prevalence of essential tremor: door-to-door neurologic exams in Mersin Province, Turkey. Neurology. 2003;61:1804–6.
10. Louis ED, Marder K, Cote L, et al. Differences in the prevalence of essential tremor among elderly African Americans, whites, and Hispanics in northern Manhattan, NY. Arch Neurol. 1995;52:1201–5.
11. Louis ED, Ford B, Frucht S, Barnes LF, X-Tang M, Ottman R. Risk of tremor and impairment from tremor in relatives of patients with essential tremor: a community-based family study. Ann Neurol. 2001;49:761–9.
12. Gulcher JR, Jonsson P, Kong A, et al. Mapping of a familial essential tremor gene, FET1, to chromosome 3q13. Nat Genet. 1997;17:84–7.
13. Higgins JJ, Pho LT, Nee LE. A gene (ETM) for essential tremor maps to chromosome 2p22-p25. Mov Disord. 1997;12:859–64.
14. Merner ND, Girard SL, Catoire H, et al. Exome sequencing identifies FUS mutations as a cause of essential tremor. Am J Hum Genet. 2012;91:313–9.
15. Shatunov A, Sambuughin N, Jankovic J, et al. Genomewide scans in North American families reveal genetic linkage of essential tremor to a region on chromosome 6p23. Brain. 2006;129:2318–31.
16. Kuhlenbaumer G, Hopfner F, Deuschl G. Genetics of essential tremor: meta-analysis and review. Neurology. 2014;82:1000–7.
17. Louis ED. Environmental epidemiology of essential tremor. Neuroepidemiology. 2008;31:139–49.
18. Tanner CM, Goldman SM, Lyons KE, et al. Essential tremor in twins: an assessment of genetic vs environmental determinants of etiology. Neurology. 2001;57:1389–91.

19. Louis ED, Factor-Litvak P, Liu X, et al. Elevated brain harmane (1-methyl-9H-pyrido[3,4-b]indole) in essential tremor cases vs. controls. Neurotoxicology. 2013;38:131–5.

20. Louis ED, Jiang W, Pellegrino KM, et al. Elevated blood harmane (1-methyl-9H-pyrido[3,4-b]indole) concentrations in essential tremor. Neurotoxicology. 2008;29:294–300.

21. Growdon JH, Shahani BT, Young RR. The effect of alcohol on essential tremor. Neurology. 1975;25:259–62.

22. Pahwa R, Lyons KE, Wilkinson SB, et al. Comparison of thalamotomy to deep brain stimulation of the thalamus in essential tremor. Mov Disord. 2001;16:140–3.

23. Raethjen J, Deuschl G. The oscillating central network of essential tremor. Clin Neurophysiol. 2012;123:61–4.

24. Kralic JE, Criswell HE, Osterman JL, et al. Genetic essential tremor in gamma-aminobutyric acidA receptor alpha1 subunit knockout mice. J Clin Invest. 2005;115:774–9.

25. Elias WJ, Huss D, Voss T, et al. A pilot study of focused ultrasound thalamotomy for essential tremor. N Engl J Med. 2013;369:640–8.

26. Schuurman PR, Bosch DA, Bossuyt PM, et al. A comparison of continuous thalamic stimulation and thalamotomy for suppression of severe tremor. N Engl J Med. 2000;342:461–8.

27. Hua SE, Lenz FA. Posture-related oscillations in human cerebellar thalamus in essential tremor are enabled by voluntary motor circuits. J Neurophysiol. 2005;93:117–27.

28. Koller WC, Lyons KE, Wilkinson SB, Troster AI, Pahwa R. Long-term safety and efficacy of unilateral deep brain stimulation of the thalamus in essential tremor. Mov Disord. 2001;16:464–8.

29. Louis ED, Babij R, Lee M, Cortes E, Vonsattel JP. Quantification of cerebellar hemispheric purkinje cell linear density: 32 ET cases versus 16 controls. Mov Disord. 2013;28:1854–9.

30. Louis ED, Faust PL, Vonsattel JP, et al. Neuropathological changes in essential tremor: 33 cases compared with 21 controls. Brain. 2007;130:3297–307.

31. Symanski C, Shill HA, Dugger B, et al. Essential tremor is not associated with cerebellar Purkinje cell loss. Mov Disord. 2014;29:496–500.

32. Rajput AH, Robinson CA, Rajput ML, Rajput A. Cerebellar Purkinje cell loss is not pathognomonic of essential tremor. Parkinsonism Relat Disord. 2011;17:16–21.

33. Chou KL. In the clinic. Parkinson disease. Ann Intern Med. 2012;157:ITC5-1–ITC5-16.

34. Louis ED, Rios E. Embarrassment in essential tremor: prevalence, clinical correlates and therapeutic implications. Parkinsonism Relat Disord. 2009;15:535–8.
35. Elble RJ, Higgins C, Leffler K, Hughes L. Factors influencing the amplitude and frequency of essential tremor. Mov Disord. 1994;9:589–96.
36. Findley LJ, Gresty MA, Halmagyi GM. Tremor, the cogwheel phenomenon and clonus in Parkinson's disease. J Neurol Neurosurg Psychiatry. 1981;44:534–46.
37. Elble RJ. Essential tremor frequency decreases with time. Neurology. 2000;55:1547–51.
38. Calzetti S, Baratti M, Gresty M, Findley L. Frequency/amplitude characteristics of postural tremor of the hands in a population of patients with bilateral essential tremor: implications for the classification and mechanism of essential tremor. J Neurol Neurosurg Psychiatry. 1987;50:561–7.
39. Rocca WA, Bower JH, Ahlskog JE, et al. Increased risk of essential tremor in first-degree relatives of patients with Parkinson's disease. Mov Disord. 2007;22:1607–14.
40. Tan EK, Lee SS, Fook-Chong S, Lum SY. Evidence of increased odds of essential tremor in Parkinson's disease. Mov Disord. 2008;23:993–7.
41. Benito-Leon J, Louis ED, Bermejo-Pareja F, Neurological Disorders in Central Spain Study Group. Risk of incident Parkinson's disease and parkinsonism in essential tremor: a population based study. J Neurol Neurosurg Psychiatry. 2009;80:423–5.
42. Geraghty JJ, Jankovic J, Zetusky WJ. Association between essential tremor and Parkinson's disease. Ann Neurol. 1985;17:329–33.
43. Rana AQ, Boke BN, Qureshi AR, Rana MA, Rahman M. Prevalence of essential tremor in an idiopathic Parkinson's disease patient population. Int J Neurosci. 2014. doi:10.3109/00207454.2014.929128.
44. Louis ED, Dogu O. Isolated head tremor: part of the clinical spectrum of essential tremor? Data from population-based and clinic-based case samples. Mov Disord. 2009;24:2281–5.
45. Louis ED, Pellegrino KM, Rios E. Unawareness of head tremor in essential tremor: a study of three samples of essential tremor patients. Mov Disord. 2008;23:2423–4.
46. Sulica L, Louis ED. Clinical characteristics of essential voice tremor: a study of 34 cases. Laryngoscope. 2010;120:516–28.

47. Louis ED, Rios E, Applegate LM, Hernandez NC, Andrews HF. Jaw tremor: prevalence and clinical correlates in three essential tremor case samples. Mov Disord. 2006;21:1872–8.

48. Fasano A, Herzog J, Raethjen J, et al. Gait ataxia in essential tremor is differentially modulated by thalamic stimulation. Brain. 2010;133:3635–48.

49. Stolze H, Petersen G, Raethjen J, Wenzelburger R, Deuschl G. The gait disorder of advanced essential tremor. Brain. 2001;124:2278–86.

50. Helmchen C, Hagenow A, Miesner J, et al. Eye movement abnormalities in essential tremor may indicate cerebellar dysfunction. Brain. 2003;126:1319–32.

51. Chandran V, Pal PK. Essential tremor: beyond the motor features. Parkinsonism Relat Disord. 2012;18:407–13.

52. Gasparini M, Bonifati V, Fabrizio E, et al. Frontal lobe dysfunction in essential tremor: a preliminary study. J Neurol. 2001;248:399–402.

53. Troster AI, Woods SP, Fields JA, et al. Neuropsychological deficits in essential tremor: an expression of cerebello-thalamo-cortical pathophysiology? Eur J Neurol. 2002;9:143–51.

54. Benito-Leon J, Louis ED, Bermejo-Pareja F, Neurological Disorders in Central Spain Study Group. Elderly-onset essential tremor is associated with dementia. Neurology. 2006;66:1500–5.

55. Thawani SP, Schupf N, Louis ED. Essential tremor is associated with dementia: prospective population-based study in New York. Neurology. 2009;73:621–5.

56. Chatterjee A, Jurewicz EC, Applegate LM, Louis ED. Personality in essential tremor: further evidence of non-motor manifestations of the disease. J Neurol Neurosurg Psychiatry. 2004;75:958–61.

57. Thenganatt MA, Louis ED. Personality profile in essential tremor: a case-control study. Parkinsonism Relat Disord. 2012;18:1042–4.

58. Tan EK, Fook-Chong S, Lum SY, et al. Non-motor manifestations in essential tremor: use of a validated instrument to evaluate a wide spectrum of symptoms. Parkinsonism Relat Disord. 2005;11:375–80.

59. Louis ED, Benito-Leon J, Bermejo-Pareja F, Neurological Disorders in Central Spain Study Group. Self-reported depression and anti-depressant medication use in essential tremor: cross-sectional and prospective analyses in a population-based study. Eur J Neurol. 2007;14:1138–46.

60. Louis ED, Barnes L, Albert SM, et al. Correlates of functional disability in essential tremor. Mov Disord. 2001;16:914–20.
61. Louis ED, Benito-Leon J, Ottman R, Bermejo-Pareja F, Neurological Disorders in Central Spain Study Group. A population-based study of mortality in essential tremor. Neurology. 2007;69:1982–9.

Chapter 3
Clinical Approach to Essential Tremor

Historical Considerations

When obtaining a history, the clinician should pay attention to the points brought out in Chap. 1, namely: the positional properties of the tremor (rest vs. action) and body region affected. Remember, ET is an action tremor, typically involving the hands first [1, 2]. A positive family history and alcohol responsiveness are factors that support the diagnosis of ET, though do not need to be present for the diagnosis to be made [3].

Other considerations include the nature of tremor onset. ET tends to have a gradual onset, while an abrupt onset may signal an underlying psychogenic cause [4]. The medication list should be closely looked at for any medications that cause tremor. Finally, a careful review of systems should be conducted, focusing on ruling out symptoms that might be seen with other tremor disorders, such as parkinsonism (slowness of movement, shuffling gait, micrographia, etc.), thyroid problems (diaphoresis, tachycardia, palpitations, weight loss), or dystonia (pulling sensations or muscle contractions).

Physical Examination

In addition to a general neurological examination, the following steps may be helpful to specifically assess for essential tremor.

A.Q. Rana, K.L. Chou, *Essential Tremor in Clinical Practice*,
In Clinical Practice, DOI 10.1007/978-3-319-14598-3_3,
© Springer International Publishing Switzerland 2015

1. Asking the patient to hold arms straight outstretched, extended at elbows with fingers spread apart. See Fig. 3.1.
2. Holding arms with fingers spread apart, flexed at elbows in front of the chest (wing beating position). See Fig. 3.2.
3. With arms in the wing beating position, have the patient make a fist with both hands while leaving the index finger of each hand extended, pointing towards each other in close proximity without touching (author calls this "One to One test"). This may help assess subtle cases of postural tremor. See Fig. 3.3.
4. Finger-Nose-Finger testing.
5. Asking the patient to hold a cup, at least four inches tall, full of water (up to one inch from the top) and to bring it to their lips and then away from their mouth a few times to see if there is any spillage of water (glass test). Pouring of liquids may also be tested.

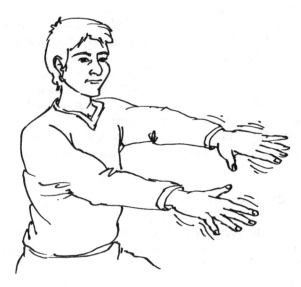

FIG. 3.1 Outstretched position of hands in postural tremor (Image courtesy of Evelyn Shifflett)

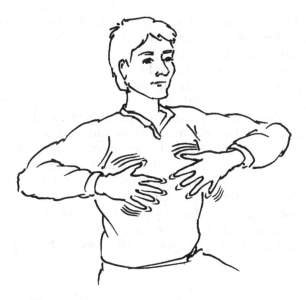

FIG. 3.2 Wing beating position of hands in postural tremor (Image courtesy of Evelyn Shifflett)

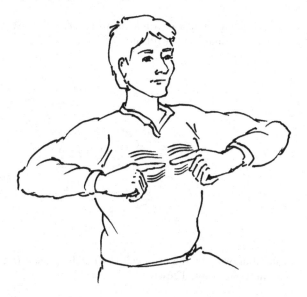

FIG. 3.3 One to one test (Image courtesy of Evelyn Shifflett)

6. Writing a standard sentence on each visit. The new writing sample on each visit is then compared to the writing sample from the previous visit in order to assess therapeutic response. See Fig. 3.4.
7. Drawing a spiral without supporting the hand on each visit and comparing the drawing to the one from previous visit in order to assess therapeutic response. See Fig. 3.5.
8. Examining for facial tremor in the half- hearted smile.
9. Determining involvement of the voice by sustained phonation and asking the patient to hold a prolonged note such as "EEEEEEEEEEEEE." Sustained phonation may also activate or increase a head tremor.
10. Inspecting the head carefully for tremor as well as for any abnormal position, such as a turn (torticollis) or tilt (laterocollis) to any side, anterocollis (forward bending) or

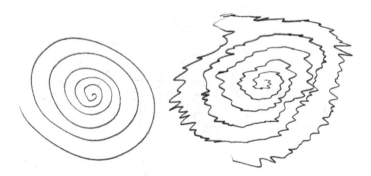

FIG. 3.4 Handwriting sample of a patient with very mild essential tremor (Today is a sunny day in Toronto)

FIG. 3.5 Spiral drawing by the examiner (*left*) and a patient (*right*) with essential tremor (Spiral Test)

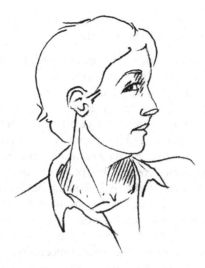

Fig. 3.6 Patient with left torticollis (Image courtesy of Evelyn Shifflett)

retrocollis (backward bending) and sagittal or lateral shift of head which may be seen in cervical dystonia. (See Fig. 3.6.) The clinician may find it helpful to inspect the patient from front, behind, as well as from each side, standing at a distance of a few feet from the patient to determine the abnormal head or neck position. Mild head tremor may be easily missed unless the head is specifically examined. Asking the patient to close their eyes for a few minutes, and allowing their head do what it likes to do may enhance the examination. Neck muscles should be inspected and palpated for any asymmetry in size if dystonic head tremor (cervical dystonia) is suspected.

11. The tongue is examined at rest in the mouth and while it is partially protruded out.

12. Lips, jaw, chin and lower extremities should also be examined for tremor. Tremor in the legs can be assessed by flexion at hips and knees with foot in dorsi-flexion.

13. To assess for features of parkinsonism, the following clinical maneuvers are suggested:

    (a) Examination for resting tremor with hands, arms and legs at complete rest supported against gravity in supine position. A latent tremor may be brought out by an activation maneuver such as saying the months of the year backwards or performing serial 7's.

    (b) Examination for rigidity, a velocity independent increase in muscle tone, by passive movements at wrists and elbows. A mild cogwheeling of upper extremities may be present in many elderly individuals but is not significant when other features of Parkinsonism are absent.

    (c) Examination for bradykinesia by fist clenching, finger tapping, rapid supination and pronation of arms and leg agility movements. Decrease in speed, drop in amplitude or early fatigue is a sign of bradykinesia. It is important to be aware that elderly essential tremor patients may have mild bradykinesia and limb rigidity as part of aging.

    (d) Examination of gait including ability to stand up from a deep seated chair. Start hesitation, base and speed of walking, stride length, arm swing, posture of trunk and turning should be observed carefully. (See Fig. 3.7.) Gait should also be observed for any freezing, which is the sudden cessation of mobility while walking. Freezing may occur at the start of walking, going through a doorway, turning, or reaching the destination. Freezing may be seen in parkinsonism and is more common in atypical parkinsonism.

    (e) Pull test for assessment of postural reflexes.

14. To assess cerebellar involvement, the following examinations are suggested:

    (a) Assessment for dysdiadochokinesia (Asking the patient to tap the palm of left hand with the palm of the right, then rapidly turn over the right hand and tap the dorsum of the right hand on the palm of the left hand, repeatedly. The same maneuver is then asked of the patient, but switching hands.)

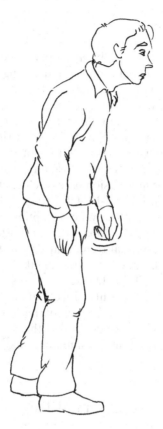

FIG. 3.7 Stooping of posture in Parkinson disease (Image courtesy of Evelyn Shifflett)

(b) Heel-Knee-Shin testing.
(c) Tandem gait testing (walking heel-to-toe). Patients with severe essential tremor may have mild difficulty with tandem gait.
(d) Assessment of speech for dysarthria and examination of extraocular movements for nystagmus. Patients with cerebellar disorders may have scanning of speech and rebound nystagmus.

Investigations

Thyroid testing should probably be performed in all patients who present with action tremor [5]. In young patients (under the age of 40) with any tremor other than mild ET or enhanced physiologic tremor, Wilson's disease should be excluded with 24 h urine copper, serum ceruloplasmin, and slit lamp examination for Kayser-Fleischer rings [6].

Brain imaging with CT or MRI is not required in typical cases of ET unless a structural cause for tremor, such as brain trauma, stroke, or mass lesion is suspected. Dopamine transporter imaging using ^{123}I-FP-CIT single photon emission tomography (DaTscan) may be an option. ^{123}I-FP-CIT is a radioligand that binds to dopamine transporters in the brain. In patients with essential tremor, uptake of this radioligand should be normal, while decreased uptake is seen in patients with parkinsonism. Thus, DaTscan can distinguish essential tremor patients from patients with dopaminergic denervation (i.e. Parkinson disease and other parkinsonian syndromes) [7]. However, evidence suggests that the diagnosis obtained from a careful history and examination may be just as good as a DaTscan.

Rating Scales for Essential Tremor

Individual clinicians use different methods to grade the tremor and follow the progress in subsequent visits after the treatment is introduced. However, there are several validated scales that can be used to document severity or progression of essential tremor. In the clinical literature, the Fahn-Tolosa-Marin scale is one of the most widely used, though it can also rate tremor in other disorders, such as orthostatic tremor, and is not specific to ET [8, 9]. The Washington Heights-Inwood Genetic Study of Essential Tremor (WHIGET) Tremor Rating Scale and the Tremor Research Group Essential Tremor Rating Assessment Scale (TETRAS) are two scales developed specifically for essential tremor [10–12].

The Fahn-Tolosa-Marin scale contains 10 items that rate tremor severity in the head, face, tongue, voice, trunk and limbs (part A), 5 items that rate tremor severity while performing activities such as writing, drawing spirals and straight lines, and pouring water between cups (Part B), and 8 items that evaluate functional disability for various daily tasks, such as feeding, drinking, working, etc. (Part C). Parts A and B are rated by clinicians while part C is largely rated by patients [9].

Of the 2 scales specifically developed for ET, TETRAS is slightly more complete. TETRAS does not take long to administer and contains both a motor and an Activities of Daily Living (ADL) subscale [10]. The ADL subscale contains 12 items pertaining to the tremor's impact on activities, such as feeding, drinking, dressing, etc. The motor subscale has 9 items rating severity of action tremor in the head, face, voice, trunk and limbs from 0 to 4 in half point intervals. The WHIGET Tremor Rating Scale on the other hand, is an examination of upper extremity tremor only. Tremor is rated at rest, with arm extension, pouring water between two cups, drinking water from a cup, using a spoon to drink water, finger-to-nose testing, and drawing spirals using a scale from 0 to 3 (except for kinetic tremor tasks which use a scale from 0 to 4) [11, 12].

References

1. Bain PG, Findley LJ, Thompson PD, et al. A study of hereditary essential tremor. Brain. 1994;117(Pt 4):805–24.
2. Lou JS, Jankovic J. Essential tremor: clinical correlates in 350 patients. Neurology. 1991;41:234–8.
3. Bain P, Brin M, Deuschl G, et al. Criteria for the diagnosis of essential tremor. Neurology. 2000;54:S7.
4. Morgante F, Edwards MJ, Espay AJ. Psychogenic movement disorders. Continuum (Minneap Minn). 2013;19:1383–96.
5. Chou KL. Diagnosis and management of the patient with tremor. Med Health R I. 2004;87:135–8.
6. Louis ED. Essential tremor. Handb Clin Neurol. 2011;100:433–48.

7. Benamer TS, Patterson J, Grosset DG, et al. Accurate differen-
   tiation of parkinsonism and essential tremor using visual assessment of [123I]-FP-CIT SPECT imaging: the [123I]-FP-CIT study
   group. Mov Disord. 2000;15:503–10.
8. Elble R, Bain P, Forjaz MJ, et al. Task force report: scales for
   screening and evaluating tremor: critique and recommendations.
   Mov Disord. 2013;28:1793–800.
9. Fahn S, Tolosa E, Marin C. Clinical rating scale for tremor. In:
   Jankovic J, Tolosa E, editors. Parkinson's disease and movement
   disorders. 2nd ed. Baltimore: Williams & Wilkins; 1993.
   p. 225–34.
10. Elble R, Comella C, Fahn S, et al. Reliability of a new scale for
    essential tremor. Mov Disord. 2012;27:1567–9.
11. Louis ED, Barnes L, Wendt KJ, et al. A teaching videotape for
    the assessment of essential tremor. Mov Disord. 2001;16:89–93.
12. Louis ED, Ottman R, Ford B, et al. The Washington Heights-
    Inwood Genetic Study of Essential Tremor: methodologic issues
    in essential-tremor research. Neuroepidemiology. 1997;16:124–33.

Chapter 4
Diagnosis of Essential Tremor

Making the Diagnosis

Several diagnostic criteria exist for the diagnosis of essential tremor (ET), but they are all similar [1–3]. All require *the presence of an action tremor in both upper extremities (kinetic or postural) in the absence of other medical conditions or drugs that cause tremor.*

On examination, patients should have an absence of other focal neurological findings except mild cogwheeling, especially in the elderly patients. Supportive (but not essential) features include positive family history of ET and tremor responsiveness to alcohol [1, 2]. Disease duration longer than 5 years without other neurologic signs also supports the diagnosis of essential tremor, but is not an absolute criterion [1, 2].

Features that would suggest another diagnosis for tremor include:

1. Presence of abnormal focal neurological findings or sensory or motor signs, especially dystonia (abnormal postures)
2. History of recent trauma before the onset of tremor
3. History of factors that may cause enhanced physiologic tremor such as hyperthyroidism
4. History of sudden onset or stepwise progression of tremor

A.Q. Rana, K.L. Chou, *Essential Tremor in Clinical Practice*, 31
In Clinical Practice, DOI 10.1007/978-3-319-14598-3_4,
© Springer International Publishing Switzerland 2015

5. Presence of wide variability in tremor frequency, give-way weakness, entrainment or distractibility (suggesting psychogenic tremor)
6. Tremor affecting only the legs (might suggest primary orthostatic tremor or Parkinson disease)
7. Isolated voice tremor
8. Isolated position-specific or task specific tremor (such as primary writing tremor).
9. Unilateral tremor of prolonged duration, unilateral leg tremor, gait dysfunction, resting tremor, bradykinesia or rigidity.
10. History of antipsychotics/antiemetics or other drug use that might cause or exacerbate tremor

Differential Diagnosis

One of the main concerns for patients who present to the clinic with a complaint of tremor is Parkinson disease, so this entity will be discussed first. With a careful history and examination, however, one should be able to distinguish ET from Parkinson disease fairly easily. (See Table 4.1 for a comparison of tremor features between ET, Parkinson disease, and enhanced physiologic tremor.) The rest of the differential diagnosis for ET includes (in alphabetical order) cerebellar tremor, drug-induced tremor, dystonic tremor, enhanced physiologic tremor, Fragile X associated tremor-ataxia syndrome (FXTAS), Holmes tremor, primary writing tremor, orthostatic tremor, and psychogenic tremor. Wilson disease would be a consideration in patients under the age of 40.

Parkinson Disease

Parkinson disease tremor classically presents as a resting tremor in a limb. The tremor diminishes with activity and posture. The frequency of Parkinson disease tremor is in the range of 3–6 Hz [4]. In the hands, the tremor is typically characterized as pill-rolling (a pronation-supination movement of

TABLE 4.1 Comparison of enhanced physiological tremor, ET and Parkinson disease tremor

	Enhanced physiological tremor	Essential tremor	Parkinson disease
Common body parts affected	Hands	Hands, head, voice	Hands or arms, legs, chin
Accompanying symptoms	None or symptoms of anxiety state	None	Rigidity, bradykinesia and postural instability
Frequency	10–14 Hz	Mainly 7–10 Hz (but may range from 4 to 12 Hz)	3–6 Hz
Positional component	Posture>Kinetic	Kinetic>posture, may have a slight resting component if severe	Resting (may have a postural/kinetic or re-emergent component in severe cases)
Symmetry	Bilateral, symmetric	Bilateral, can be mildly asymmetrical	Initially unilateral, bilateral and asymmetrical in advanced stage
Course	Usually non progressive	Progressive	Progressive
Response to alcohol	Minimal or none	Responds significantly	None
Effect of caffeine, stress, stimulants	Increases	Increases	Increases
Inheritance	None	Autosomal dominant with variable penetrance	Sporadic or related to genetics of Parkinson disease

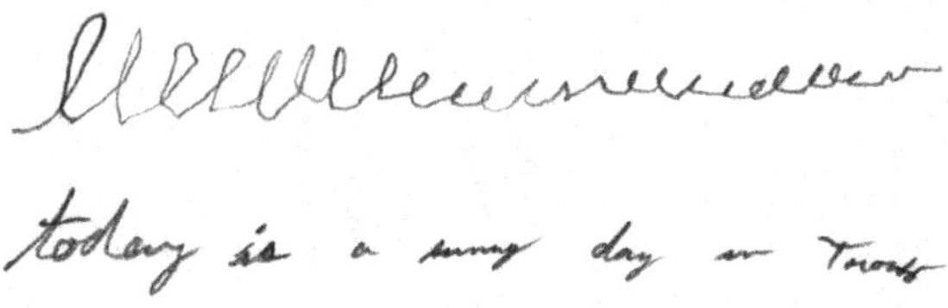

FIG. 4.1 Multiple loops and handwriting sample of a Parkinson disease patient with micrographia (Today is a sunny day in Toronto)

the wrist) [5]. Tremor in Parkinson disease typically starts unilaterally, in the hand or arm [6]. The tremor may also progress to involve the legs, and chin/lips but usually does not involve the head or voice. This type of tremor should be accompanied by other signs of Parkinson disease such as bradykinesia, rigidity and in more advanced cases, postural instability [5]. History of the other features of Parkinson disease such as drooling, difficulty with dexterity and micrographia (see Fig. 4.1) may be elicited.

Up to 93 % percent of patients with Parkinson disease may have action tremor in addition to the typical resting tremor though the action tremor typically occurs in combination with resting tremor and is much less noticeable than the resting tremor [7, 8]. Some Parkinson disease patients may have a re-emergent rest tremor. This is a postural tremor of the hands that appears with a several second latency after the hands adopt the outstretched position and has a frequency typical of the rest tremor in PD [8]. The postural tremor in ET appears immediately with upon adopting the outstretched posture position. It is an important distinction as the re-emergent rest tremor in PD may be mislabelled as an action tremor [9]. Parkinson disease is treated with dopaminergic medications.

Cerebellar Tremor

Cerebellar tremor causes a slow, coarse oscillation of the limbs at a frequency of approximately 3–5 Hz in a horizontal plane [2]. The tremor in the limbs is generated proximally.

Tremor of the head and trunk may be caused by midline cerebellar lesions. It is not a true tremor because in most cases it is ataxia of the affected limb or body part. Patients often complain of limb incoordination and gait imbalance. On exam, abnormal finger-to-nose or heel-to-shin testing, dysarthria, and a wide-based ataxic gait may be seen. Common acquired causes of cerebellar tremor include multiple sclerosis, head trauma, stroke, or cerebellar haemorrhage. A family history of cerebellar ataxia may suggest a genetic cause [10]. Cerebellar tremor is extremely difficult to treat.

Drug-Induced Tremor

Drug-induced tremors have an onset that is temporally related to the history of medication usage. The tremor is usually symmetrical and can cause pure rest tremors, pure action tremors, or a mixed rest/action tremor [11]. Though many medications have been implicated in the causation of drug induced tremors, common ones are listed in Table 4.2. It may take weeks to months for the tremor to improve after discontinuation of the offending agent.

TABLE 4.2 Most common medications that cause tremors

Anti-arrhythmics	Amiodarone
Anti-depressants/mood stabilizers	Lithium, amitriptyline, SSRIs
Anti-epileptics	Valproic acid
Antipsychotics	All typical and atypical antipsychotics can cause tremor except quetiapine and clozapine
Bronchodilators	Salbutamol
Drugs of misuse	Cocaine, ethanol, nicotine
Gastrointestinal drugs	Prochlorperazine, metoclopramide
Immunosuppressants	Tacrolimus, Cyclosporin
Methylxanthines	Caffeine

Dystonia

Dystonic Tremor is a postural and/or a kinetic tremor which is usually not seen during complete repose and occurs in a body part or limb affected by dystonia. These tremors are usually focal with irregular amplitudes. While focal limb or jaw dystonias can occur, the most common form of a focal dystonia is cervical dystonia [12]. These patients often have an irregular, rotatory head tremor accompanied by neck pain. They may find that touching certain parts of their head or face with their hand or finger may help in transiently diminishing the amplitude of the tremor. This phenomenon is known as a "sensory trick" and is helpful in establishing the diagnosis of dystonic head tremor due to cervical dystonia [2, 13, 14]. (See Fig. 4.2) Postural hand tremor may be associated with cervical dystonia in about 30 % of patients [14]. Although this condition may become apparent at any age, symptoms

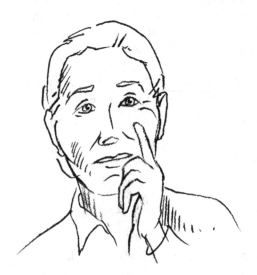

FIG. 4.2 Dystonic head tremor stops by touching the side of face (sensory trick) (Image courtesy of Evelyn Shifflett)

usually begin between the ages of 20–60 years [12]. Women are affected twice more than men [12]. Botulinum toxin is the treatment of choice for dystonic tremor.

Enhanced Physiologic Tremor

Enhanced physiologic tremor is a result of the interaction of numerous mechanical and neuromuscular influences. A physiologic tremor occurs in every person, but may not be visible to the eye. An enhanced physiologic tremor is simply an exacerbation of this normal tremor by various psychological and metabolic aggravating factors, including anxiety, fear, fatigue or exhaustion, hypoglycemia, hyperthyroidism, caffeine, alcohol withdrawal, or infection. This tremor has a frequency of 10–14 Hz. Once the identifying cause is identified and corrected, the tremor typically resolves.

Fragile X Associated Tremor-Ataxia Syndrome (FXTAS) [15, 16]

Fragile X associated tremor-ataxia syndrome (FXTAS) usually affects individuals above the age of 65 years. About two thirds of patients manifest a kinetic tremor. In fragile X syndrome and fragile X-associated tremor-ataxia syndrome, there is expansion of CGG repeats of the FMR1 gene on chromosome Xq27.3. The normal number of CGG repeats is 6–50, the carriers have 50–200 repeats, and fragile X syndrome patients have 200–1,500 repeats. The fragile X-associated tremor ataxia syndrome occurs in the carriers and has a prevalence of 1 in 3,000 men above age of 50. FXTAS patients may have an impaired gait and fine motor skills, cerebellar ataxia, fluctuating weakness, sensory symptoms, sexual dysfunction, bladder or bowel dysfunction, parkinsonism, weakness of proximal lower extremities, and cognitive dysfunction. Females with fragile X-associated tremor/ataxia syndrome have also been described contrary to previous reports.

Holmes Tremor

Holmes tremor (aka rubral or midbrain tremor) was first described by Gordon Holmes in 1904 [2]. It is an undulating tremor, and has rest, postural and kinetic components [2]. This tremor is characterized by a frequency of 2–5 Hz but has high amplitude and is extremely debilitating [2]. This tremor is likely to be caused by interruption of fibers in the superior cerebellar peduncle which carry cerebello-thalamic and cerebello-olivary projections in the midbrain contralateral to the affected limb [17]. Some of the known causes of Holmes tremor include cerebrovascular accidents, multiple sclerosis, infection, hypoxia, trauma, and cystic lesions which interrupt fibers of the superior cerebellar peduncle carrying cerebello-thalamic and cerebello-olivary projections in the midbrain. Treatment of Holmes tremor is challenging as it responds poorly to medical treatments.

Primary Writing Tremor

Primary writing tremor is characterized by its large amplitude and occurs at a frequency of 5–6 Hz [18]. This tremor only occurs during the act of writing or when the hand assumes a writing position and only involves the affected arm [2]. Primary writing tremor is often unilateral but may involve the other side in some advanced cases. This tremor may be difficult to distinguish from writer's cramp or essential tremor that is aggravated by writing. Primary writing tremor may respond to botulinum toxin or thalamic stimulation.

Orthostatic Tremor

Orthostatic tremor is typically a lower extremity tremor which occurs upon standing (usually after a short latency) and disappears with walking (involves the legs and trunk) [2]. Upper limbs, when involved, are synchronous with the lower extremities. It may cause patients to feel unsteady while standing but not while walking except in severe cases. These patients do not have a problem sitting or lying down. The diagnosis of this tremor can be confirmed by electromyographic discharges of a 14–18 Hz pattern [2, 19]. All muscles show this pattern, which is absent during sitting and lying down [2]. Presence of a coherent high-frequency electromyographic discharge pattern, in all the involved muscles, suggests that orthostatic tremor is a central tremor [19]. This tremor can be treated with clonazepam, primidone and gabapentin although the response may not be great [19].

Psychogenic Tremor

Psychogenic tremors have variable erratic frequency and fluctuations in amplitude [20]. The tremor may go into remission for variable periods of time but may recur spontaneously. Usually the frequency is 6 Hz or less. On examination, the tremor may display distractibility, where the tremor remits or stops temporarily when performing voluntary repetitive movements of another body part. Entrainment, where the frequency of the psychogenic tremor begins to correspond to the frequency of voluntary repetitive movements of another limb, may also be seen.

The following features may be helpful in diagnosing psychogenic tremor [20]:

1. Abrupt onset of symptoms.
2. Spontaneous episodes of symptom remission with a fluctuating course.
3. Variability of phenomenology and severity over time.
4. Characteristics that do not fit with recognized physiological patterns such as entrainment, increase with attention or decrease with distraction.
5. Presence of other features suggestive of a conversion disorder such as give-way weakness, false sensory signs, rhythmical shaking, deliberate slowness in carrying out voluntary movement and excessive startle in response to sudden, unexpected noise or threatening movement.
6. Resolution of symptoms in response to placebo, suggestion or psychotherapy.

Psychological or psychiatric disturbances do not need to be present for the diagnosis of a psychogenic tremor to be made. The authors prefer not to treat these patients with tremor medications. Non-pharmacologic approaches, including cognitive behavioural therapy and physical therapy may be helpful. If depression and anxiety are present, referral to a psychiatrist may also be helpful.

Wilson Disease

Wilson disease is one of the few movement disorders that is curable. It is an inborn error of copper metabolism causing liver abnormalities and basal ganglia damage. It is autosomal recessive and the gene responsible encodes for a copper-transporting ATP-ase. Mutations in this gene cause a failure of copper excretion from the liver, leading to buildup of copper in the liver and other sites, such as the brain. It may cause any number of neurologic problems, including tremor, dysarthria, incoordination, dystonia, gait abnormalities. The tremor of Wilson disease is commonly characterized as a wing-beating tremor [21]. The diagnosis may be made with detection of a low serum ceruloplasmin in combination with high urinary copper excretion. Virtually all patients with neurologic manifestations of Wilson disease have Kayser-Fleischer rings upon careful slit lamp examination [21]. D-penicillamine is the treatment of choice.

References

1. Bain P, Brin M, Deuschl G, et al. Criteria for the diagnosis of essential tremor. Neurology. 2000;54:S7.
2. Deuschl G, Bain P, Brin M. Consensus statement of the Movement Disorder Society on tremor. Ad Hoc Scientific Committee. Mov Disord. 1998;13 Suppl 3:2–23.
3. Louis ED, Ottman R, Ford B, et al. The Washington Heights-Inwood Genetic Study of Essential Tremor: methodologic issues in essential-tremor research. Neuroepidemiology. 1997;16:124–33.

4. Findley LJ, Gresty MA, Halmagyi GM. Tremor, the cogwheel phenomenon and clonus in Parkinson's disease. J Neurol Neurosurg Psychiatry. 1981;44:534–46.
5. Chou KL. In the clinic. Parkinson disease. Ann Intern Med. 2012;157:ITC5-1–ITC5-16.
6. Hughes AJ, Daniel SE, Lees AJ. The clinical features of Parkinson's disease in 100 histologically proven cases. Adv Neurol. 1993;60:595–9.
7. Koller WC, Vetere-Overfield B, Barter R. Tremors in early Parkinson's disease. Clin Neuropharmacol. 1989;12:293–7.
8. Louis ED, Levy G, Cote LJ, Mejia H, Fahn S, Marder K. Clinical correlates of action tremor in Parkinson disease. Arch Neurol. 2001;58:1630–4.
9. Jain S, Lo SE, Louis ED. Common misdiagnosis of a common neurological disorder: how are we misdiagnosing essential tremor? Arch Neurol. 2006;63:1100–4.
10. Schols L, Bauer P, Schmidt T, Schulte T, Riess O. Autosomal dominant cerebellar ataxias: clinical features, genetics, and pathogenesis. Lancet Neurol. 2004;3:291–304.
11. Morgan JC, Sethi KD. Drug-induced tremors. Lancet Neurol. 2005;4:866–76.
12. Stacy M. Epidemiology, clinical presentation, and diagnosis of cervical dystonia. Neurol Clin. 2008;26 Suppl 1:23–42.
13. Jahanshahi M. Factors that ameliorate or aggravate spasmodic torticollis. J Neurol Neurosurg Psychiatry. 2000;68:227–9.
14. Jankovic J, Leder S, Warner D, Schwartz K. Cervical dystonia: clinical findings and associated movement disorders. Neurology. 1991;41:1088–91.
15. Berry-Kravis E, Abrams L, Coffey SM, et al. Fragile X-associated tremor/ataxia syndrome: clinical features, genetics, and testing guidelines. Mov Disord. 2007;22:2018–30, quiz 2140.
16. Jacquemont S, Hagerman RJ, Leehey M, et al. Fragile X premutation tremor/ataxia syndrome: molecular, clinical, and neuroimaging correlates. Am J Hum Genet. 2003;72:869–78.
17. Ohye C, Shibazaki T, Hirai T, et al. A special role of the parvocellular red nucleus in lesion-induced spontaneous tremor in monkeys. Behav Brain Res. 1988;28:241–3.
18. Rana AQ, Vaid HM. A review of primary writing tremor. Int J Neurosci. 2012;122:114–8.
19. Sander HW, Masdeu JC, Tavoulareas G, Walters A, Zimmerman T, Chokroverty S. Orthostatic tremor: an electrophysiological analysis. Mov Disord. 1998;13:735–8.

20. Morgante F, Edwards MJ, Espay AJ. Psychogenic movement disorders. Continuum (Minneap Minn). 2013;19:1383–96.
21. Lorincz MT. Recognition and treatment of neurologic Wilson's disease. Semin Neurol. 2012;32:538–43.

Chapter 5
Treatment of Essential Tremor

Non-pharmacologic Treatment

Not all patients need to be started on medications. Some patients with ET may desire nothing more than to be assured that they do not have Parkinson disease. Others may decide that the tremors are not disabling enough to take medications. Any exacerbating factors, if present, should be addressed first. Tremor-inducing medications should be discontinued (see Chap. 4 for frequent drugs that induce tremors). The avoidance of stimulants such as caffeine may be helpful. Metabolic problems, such as hyperthyroidism, should also be looked for and treated [1].

Because alcohol may transiently reduce tremor amplitude in about 50–75 % of the cases [2–4], some patients may drink a glass of wine or beer at social events in order to calm down their tremors. These patients may notice a worsened tremor (rebound tremor) when the effect of alcohol wears off [4]. In general though, increased alcohol intake is not recommended for treatment of essential tremor.

Stress reduction may be helpful, though may not be easily achieved. There is no evidence that physical therapy interventions improve tremor. Cooling the upper limbs in cold water for about 5 min causes temporary reduction in essential tremor, but there are no data on the length of effectiveness of this technique over 30 min, and this technique may be too uncomfortable for most patients [5].

A.Q. Rana, K.L. Chou, *Essential Tremor in Clinical Practice*, In Clinical Practice, DOI 10.1007/978-3-319-14598-3_5, © Springer International Publishing Switzerland 2015

Non-invasive Devices

Non-invasive devices such as weighted utensils or weighted wrist bracelets are often suggested. Unfortunately, there is only limited evidence that weights reduce action tremor [5]. It is the author's experience that weights are most helpful for mild essential tremor, and that only some patients find it beneficial.

Tremor suppressing orthoses have been studied [6, 7]. These devices detect tremors from voluntary motion and use loading approaches to suppress pathologic tremors, but they are not readily available to the public. Furthermore, they may cause a lot of discomfort, and the bulk, weight, and structure of the device is likely to prevent widespread acceptance.

A handheld, non-invasive device (Liftware http://www.liftlabsdesign.com/, see Fig. 5.1) that can stabilize a spoon for eating has been recently developed [8]. This device senses the direction of a person's tremor and moves the spoon in the opposite direction in order to stabilize the spoon. It reduces tremor amplitude by about 70 % with eating tasks when tested in individuals with ET [8]. The device is light and contains a rechargeable battery that can last for several meals.

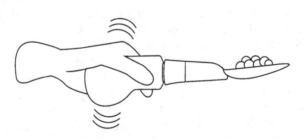

FIG. 5.1 Liftware device showing stabilization of a spoon despite tremor in the hand (Illustration by John Redmond)

Pharmacologic Treatment

Two medications are considered first-line treatment for ET: propranolol (a beta-blocker) and primidone (a GABA agonist) [9–11]. After these two agents, others, such as topiramate, gabapentin, other beta-blockers, and benzodiazepines may be tried (see Table 5.1 for a summary of medications used for ET) [10, 11]. Pharmacological treatments are generally considered to be effective in 50 % of patients with essential tremor [9, 12]. Additionally, many patients have difficulty tolerating these medications [12].

Propranolol

Propranolol use for essential tremor was introduced in 1971 [13]. Among the different beta-blockers, none is considered to be superior to propranolol [9–11]. The mechanism of action of beta-blockers in ET involves antagonism of peripheral beta-adrenergic receptors in muscles, so drugs that are predominantly central acting *B-1* antagonists appear to be less effective than those that act predominantly on peripheral *B-2* receptors [14, 15]. Propranolol is a nonselective beta-adrenergic receptor antagonist. Some patients may take propranolol only before social engagements whereas others may use it on a daily basis. If propranolol is to be taken on daily basis, the dosage ranges from 60 to 320 mg, divided into two to three doses per day [9, 11]. Propranolol is effective in treating essential tremor involving limbs, and many studies have shown that the magnitude of tremor is reduced by at least 50 % as measured by accelerometry and clinical rating scales [9, 10].

Side effects include a drop in blood pressure, fatigue, depression, impotence and bradycardia. Propranolol is contraindicated in patients with severe asthma, COPD or heart failure. Diabetes mellitus is also a relative contraindication as propranolol can mask symptoms of hypoglycemia.

TABLE 5.1 Pharmacological agents used in the treatment of essential tremor

Drug	Dose	Side effects	Comments
Primidone	Starting dose is 25 mg daily, increased slowly up to total dose 750 mg daily	Sedation, fatigue, drowsiness, nausea, vomiting, malaise and dizziness	GABA agonist
Propranolol	Starting dose is 20 mg three times daily, increased slowly up to total dose 320 mg daily	Lightheadedness, bradycardia, drowsiness, impotence, fatigue, depression	B1 & B2 antagonist
Propranolol LA	Starting dose is 60 mg once daily, increased slowly up to 320 mg/day	Skin rash, lightheadedness and dizziness	Same as propranolol but long acting
Topiramate	Starting dose is 25 mg once daily, increased weekly by 25 mg to the maximum dose of 200 mg twice daily	Weight loss, paresthesias, concentration difficulties, exacerbation of glaucoma and renal stones	Sodium channel blocker
Gabapentin	Starting dose is 300 mg once daily, increased over few days to 300–900 mg three times daily	Fatigue, dizziness, nervousness, lethargy	Alpha-2-delta calcium channel subunit blocker
Atenolol	Starting dose is 50 mg once daily, maximum 150 mg/day	Lightheadedness, nausea, cough, dry mouth, sleepiness	B1 antagonist
Sotalol	80 mg twice daily	Blurred vision, shortness of breath, lightheadedness	B1 & B2 antagonist, acting mainly peripherally

Alprazolam	Starting dose is 0.25 mg three times daily, increased slowly up to 1 mg three times daily	Fatigue, drowsiness, abuse potential	Benzodiazepine
Clonazepam	Starting dose is 0.5 mg once daily, increased slowly to 2 mg three times daily	Lethargy	Benzodiazepine
Nadolol	Starting dose is 40 mg once daily, maximum 240 mg/day	Dizziness	$B1$ & $B2$ antagonist
Nimodipine	Starting dose is 30 mg once daily, increased slowly to maximum 120 mg/day divided three times daily	Headaches and heartburn	Ca channel blocker
Botulinum toxin A for head tremor	Dose ranges from 50 to 400 units depending upon the muscles involved and degree of tremor	Excessive weakness of injected muscles, dysphagia, injection pain	Injected every 3–4 months
Botulinum toxin A for hand tremor	Dose is variable, from 50 to 100 Units/arm	Hand and finger weakness, pain at injection site	Injected every 3–4 months
Botulinum toxin A for voice tremor	0.5–15 Units	Hypophonia, dysphagia	Injected every 3–4 months

Propranolol also comes in a long acting formulation, *Propranolol LA*, that may be taken once a day. On average, Propranolol LA results in a 30–38 % improvement in limb tremor when measured by accelerometry [16, 17].

Primidone

Primidone, originally used as an antiepileptic medication, improves tremor significantly in patients with ET. Primidone acts by enhancing GABAergic tone in the central nervous system. It comes in 50 mg and 250 mg formulations. The initial dose is half of a 50 mg tablet (25 mg) which is then titrated slowly upwards. The average reduction in tremor is at least 50 % when measured by the clinical rating scales and accelerometry [10]. Though similar in effectiveness to propranolol, tolerance is an issue with primidone [9, 12]. One third of the patients may have a strong feeling of being unwell with the first dose that may be so strong that patients refuse to continue on primidone [9]. However, these side effects may improve with longer exposure. Other common side effects include drowsiness, dysequilibrium and dizziness. Because of the drowsiness, patients may tolerate it better if given at bedtime.

Combined Primidone/Propranolol

Combined treatment with propranolol and primidone may possibly be more effective than monotherapy with either of these agents alone, probably because of their different mechanisms of action. In one study, primidone, at doses of 50–1,000 mg/day decreased tremor amplitude in ET by 60–70 % when added to propranolol, compared to only a 35 % reduction in tremor with propranolol only (mean dose of 260 mg/day) [18]. Unfortunately, this issue has not been studied in a randomized, controlled fashion.

Other Therapies

Topiramate is a sodium channel blocker whose common indications include epilepsy and prophylaxis of migraine. Topiramate has been studied in three double-blind, placebo-controlled, crossover studies, and improves tremor severity, motor task performance, and functional disability, as measured by the clinical rating scales, by approximately 30 % [19]. The initial starting dose of topiramate is 25 mg once a day, but the mean dosage in these trials was approximately 250 mg a day, divided into two daily doses. Side effects include decrease in appetite, weight loss, paresthesias, concentration difficulties, exacerbation of glaucoma and renal stone.

Gabapentin may have a mild beneficial effect on essential tremor. In one double-blind, placebo-controlled, crossover trial in 16 patients, gabapentin at a dose of 1,200 mg/day had similar tremor effect to propranolol, and both were better than placebo in all tremor measures (clinical and accelerometry) [20]. In another double-blind, placebo-controlled, crossover trial using gabapentin as adjunctive therapy in ET, tremor rating scores improved, but accelerometry scores did not improve [21]. A separate, double-blind, placebo-controlled, crossover trial of gabapentin as adjunctive therapy reported no difference between placebo and gabapentin at a dose of 1,800 mg/day [22]. The side effects of gabapentin include fatigue, dizziness, nervousness and lethargy.

As mentioned above, other beta-blockers may also be used, though none are considered as good as propranolol. *Atenolol* results in approximately 25 % mean improvement on clinical tremor rating scales and a 37 % improvement by accelerometry [10, 23]. Clinically effective doses range between 50 and 150 mg per day. Side effects are similar to propranolol and include lightheadedness, nausea, cough, dry mouth and sleepiness. *Nadolol,* at a dose of 120–240 mg daily, has been demonstrated to improve tremor in ET, but only in patients who previously responded to propranolol [24].

Sotalol is another nonselective beta-adrenergic receptor antagonist that was shown to effectively reduce tremor in a double-blind placebo-controlled trial at a dose of 80 mg twice daily [15].

Benzodiazepines may be helpful for essential tremor. In small, double-blind studies, *alprazolam* has demonstrated benefit for limb tremor in ET that is superior to placebo [25] and equivalent to primidone [26]. The dose range for alprazolam is 0.75–3 mg/day. Use of alprazolam is cautioned due to its abusive potential [10]. Side effects include lightheadedness, nausea, cough, dry mouth and sleepiness. *Clonazepam* decreased tremor by about 71 % in a small study of 14 patients with kinetic limb tremor due to ET [27]. Effective doses for clonazepam range from 0.5 to 6 mg/day. Side effects include drowsiness. Similar to alprazolam, there is also potential for abuse and possibility of withdrawal symptoms associated with clonazepam, and therefore it should be used with great caution [10].

Nimodipine may potentially benefit patients with limb tremor. In one small study looking at 30 mg four times daily, 8/16 ET patients who had never been treated with other medications noticed improvement in their tremor [28]. The side effects include headache and heartburn. *Pregabalin* and *zonisamide* may also be helpful, though the literature has reported mixed results, with some studies showing effectiveness in ET, while others show no difference from placebo [10].

Botulinum toxin has been used to treat hand, head and voice tremor in essential tremor. It can improve postural hand tremor by about 50–68 %, but the incidence of finger or wrist weakness is high (approximately 70–90 % of patients) [29, 30]. For head tremor, there has been only one randomized trial. In this trial, five subjects had moderate to marked improvement in head tremor on clinical rating scales compared to only one subject with improvement who was given placebo [31]. The side effects included pain at the injection site and weakness. There have been two open label studies of botulinum toxin type A for voice tremor [32, 33].

In one study, about a 22 % improvement with unilateral injections and a 30 % improvement with bilateral injections was noticed in voice tremor [33]. In the other study, 67 % of the patients subjectively felt that their voice was improved [32]. When used to treat voice tremor, botulinum toxin may cause hoarseness of voice and swallowing difficulties. At this point, botulinum toxin injections for limb, head and voice tremor should be considered only in medically refractory cases [10, 11].

Surgical Treatment

Surgical treatment should be considered for a patient with essential tremor when: (1) the tremors are disabling and interfere with a patient's quality of life and (2) the tremors do not respond to standard medical therapies. Dementia is a contraindication to surgical procedures. Surgical centers typically do not consider potential candidates until they have failed the first-line therapies propranolol and primidone. A common mistake is marking a tremor medication as "failed" when the medication was not titrated to a high enough dose (see Table 5.1 for maximal doses of the commonly used tremor medications). Thus, prior to surgery, patients should be evaluated by a movement disorders specialist. Two types of surgical treatments are available; *deep brain stimulation (DBS) and thalamotomy* (see Table 5.2 for a comparison of surgical treatments).

Deep Brain Stimulation (DBS)

DBS for ET involves the placement of an electrode into the ventralis intermedialis (Vim) nucleus of the thalamus. The electrode is then connected via an extension wire to an implantable pulse generator (IPG) (see Fig. 5.2). The DBS procedure has advantages over lesioning treatments such as thalamotomy in that no parts of the brain are destroyed,

TABLE 5.2 Surgical treatments for essential tremor

Technique	Side effects	Comments
Deep brain stimulation of the thalamus	Due to procedure: intracranial hemorrhage, stroke Hardware malfunction Due to stimulation: dysarthria, paresthesias, dystonia, postural instability, ataxia, and limb weakness	Marked improvement in limb tremor, insufficient evidence for voice and head tremor, side effects are less than thalamotomy
Conventional thalamotomy	Transient contralateral weakness, dysarthria, contralateral hemiparesis, verbal or cognitive deficits and confusion	Marked improvement of contralateral tremor. Bilateral procedure not recommended
Gamma knife thalamotomy	Transient contralateral arm weakness and numbness, possible progressive dysarthria, dystonia of the contralateral arm and leg, and choreoathetosis	Delay before onset of improvement. Insufficient evidence
MRI-guided focused ultrasound thalamotomy	Transient paresthesias and unsteadiness. Some may have sustained paresthesias	Currently considered investigational

making the procedure reversible [34, 35]. Additionally, stimulation can be increased over time as the disease progresses. The final selection of a DBS candidate for ET should be based on a multidisciplinary evaluation, which ideally includes a movement disorders neurologist, a neurosurgeon, and a neuropsychologist. Psychiatry, speech and swallowing, and social work evaluations may also be performed prior to offering DBS surgery to a potential candidate.

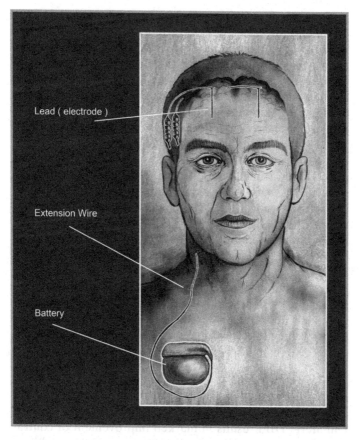

Fɪɢ. 5.2 Deep brain stimulation system (Illustration by Chris Winters)

DBS Procedure

DBS is typically performed unilaterally for ET, as bilateral Vim nucleus stimulation may cause speech problems [36]. The Vim nucleus contralateral to the patient's dominant hand is targeted. Depending on the institution where DBS is performed, electrophysiological techniques such as microelectrode recording can be used to ensure accurate placement. Microelectrode recording involves recording individual cell activity unique to specific brain structures, thus identifying the thalamus along the electrode tract [37]. Once the target location is identified, the DBS lead can be placed and macroelectrode stimulation testing can be done. (Some centers may skip microelectrode recording altogether). The purpose of macroelectrode stimulation is to check for benefits and side effects intraoperatively in order to determine proper placement. If macroelectrode stimulation causes side effects at low stimulation settings, the DBS lead may be repositioned. The DBS lead is then secured to the skull using a plastic cap to cover the Burr hole and the lead is connected via an extension wire to the IPG, all of which is implanted underneath the skin surface. The IPG is secured in a subcutaneous pocket below the clavicle overlying the chest wall. Some centers may do the entire procedure in 1 day, while others may implant the DBS lead on 1 day and implant the IPG and extension wires days to weeks later. The IPG is typically activated a few weeks after surgery to allow for any brain swelling to resolve, and post-operative programming is carried out on multiple visits over the following months.

DBS Outcomes

Unilateral DBS results in marked improvement of contra-lateral postural and kinetic limb tremor, on the order of 60–90 % [38–40]. This improvement can be maintained long-term for many years [38, 40]. Improvement in disability and quality of life also occurs after DBS and can be maintained long-term [41, 42]. Head tremor sometimes improves, but voice tremor usually does not improve with unilateral thalamic DBS [43, 44]. Bilateral Vim stimulation may be more effective for these midline tremors, but the results are inconsistent and patients may also have more dysarthria and gait difficulty [44].

Risks and Side Effects of DBS

There are 3 types of DBS-related risks or complications: those related to surgery, those related to the device, and those related to stimulation. In addition to risks common in all neurosurgical procedures, such as pulmonary embolism, pneumonia, wound infection, postoperative seizures, and perioperative confusion, DBS surgery is also associated with ~3 % chance of intracerebral haemorrhage or stroke, but typically less than 1 % of cases are associated with a neurologic deficit [45]. Cognition overall does not change with DBS for ET. Hardware-related complications may occur in up to 9 % of patients undergoing DBS, and include electrode or wire break, IPG malfunction, skin erosion and lead migration [46]. All patients with deep brain stimulation devices should be warned to avoid diathermy treatment and non-cranial MRIs, as they can lead to brain damage by heating of the electrodes.

Stimulation-related side effects of Vim DBS include dysarthria, paresthesias, dystonia, postural instability, ataxia, and limb weakness [47, 48]. These effects are noted more frequently with bilateral compared to unilateral stimulation. Many of these effects can be reduced or resolved by adjusting the stimulus parameters, but at the expense of reduced tremor suppression.

Thalamotomy

Thalamotomy is a lesioning procedure, meaning that a precise, but tiny portion of thalamic tissue is destroyed. Conventional thalamotomy has essentially been replaced by DBS at most centers because DBS appears to have fewer adverse effects. However, a couple of "non-invasive" thalamotomy techniques have been developed which can create brain lesions without surgical incisions.

Thalamotomy Procedures

Conventional surgical thalamotomy employs stereotactic and electrophysiological techniques similar to the DBS procedure to locate the place in the thalamus. Unlike DBS, lesions are then surgically created in that precise spot. Gamma-knife therapy and MRI-guided focused ultrasound are two techniques that can accomplish the same thing, but "non-invasively". For gamma-knife therapy, MRI of the head is performed and used to locate the Vim nucleus. On the day of surgery, radiation is delivered via focused beams that converge at the Vim to destroy cells [49, 50]. MRI-guided focused ultrasound is similar to gamma-knife therapy, but uses focused ultrasound beams instead of radiation to make the lesion [51]. Gamma-knife therapy and focused ultrasound thalamotomy are currently considered unproven treatments [10]. They are "non-invasive" because no incision is made and no anesthesia is given, but there is still destruction of brain tissue. They are also performed on an outpatient basis and do not require hospitalization.

Thalamotomy Outcomes

Conventional unilateral thalamotomy is very effective for the treatment of contralateral limb tremor. Open label trials have shown contralateral limb tremor reduction on the order of 80–90 %, and there is some evidence that the effects can be long lasting [52–54]. Bilateral thalamotomy results in significant dysarthria, dysphonia, and mental confusion, so it is no longer used for ET [10].

Studies of gamma-knife thalamotomy have reported that between 75 and 90 % of patients become tremor free [10]. However, patients do not typically notice improvement until weeks after the procedure (median 6 weeks), and it may take months to notice an effect [55]. Some patients may not be willing to wait that long to see results.

There has only been one uncontrolled study of MRI-guided focused ultrasound in patients with ET [51]. It involved only 15 patients, and at 1 year, contralateral hand tremor severity was reduced by 75 % and disability was improved by 85 %. Again, MRI-guided focused ultrasound is still considered investigational, and more studies will be needed before this technique is accepted as a standard treatment for ET.

Risks of Thalamotomy

In addition to typical neurosurgical risks, adverse events reported with conventional thalamotomy include permanent hemiparesis and dysarthria [34, 35, 52–54]. Other transient problems may occur, including speech and motor dysfunction, confusion and somnolence [34, 35, 52–54]. Reported complications from gamma-knife therapy include transient limb weakness and paresthesias [10, 50, 55]. However, there was one case report where the patient had progressive neurologic deficits such as numbness, dysarthria, dystonia, and choreo-athetosis, 7 months after the procedure [56]. Adverse effects of MRI-guided focused ultrasound included transient paresthesias and unsteadiness/ataxia; four patients had persistent paresthesia [51]. Larger controlled trials are planned to determine the long-term effectiveness and safety of this potentially promising procedure.

Thalamotomy vs. DBS

Based on current evidence, both conventional thalamotomy and DBS effectively treat limb tremor, but DBS has fewer adverse events than thalamotomy [10]. Other factors, such as age, medical comorbidities, and access to DBS centers may influence the decision to perform thalamotomy versus DBS. There is insufficient evidence to recommend gamma-knife or MRI-guided focused ultrasound thalamotomy at this time [10].

References

1. Louis ED. Essential tremor. Handb Clin Neurol. 2011;100: 433–48.
2. Koller WC, Busenbark K, Miner K. The relationship of essential tremor to other movement disorders: report on 678 patients. Essential Tremor Study Group. Ann Neurol. 1994;35:717–23.
3. Lou JS, Jankovic J. Essential tremor: clinical correlates in 350 patients. Neurology. 1991;41:234–8.
4. Bain PG, Findley LJ, Thompson PD, et al. A study of hereditary essential tremor. Brain. 1994;117(Pt 4):805–24.
5. O'Connor RJ, Kini MU. Non-pharmacological and non-surgical interventions for tremor: a systematic review. Parkinsonism Relat Disord. 2011;17:509–15.
6. Rocon E, Belda-Lois JM, Ruiz AF, Manto M, Moreno JC, Pons JL. Design and validation of a rehabilitation robotic exoskeleton for tremor assessment and suppression. IEEE Trans Neural Syst Rehabil Eng. 2007;15:367–78.
7. Rocon E, Manto M, Pons J, Camut S, Belda JM. Mechanical suppression of essential tremor. Cerebellum. 2007;6:73–8.
8. Pathak A, Redmond JA, Allen M, Chou KL. A noninvasive handheld assistive device to accommodate essential tremor: a pilot study. Mov Disord. 2014;29:838–42.
9. Deuschl G, Raethjen J, Hellriegel H, Elble R. Treatment of patients with essential tremor. Lancet Neurol. 2011;10:148–61.
10. Zesiewicz TA, Elble R, Louis ED, et al. Practice parameter: therapies for essential tremor: report of the Quality Standards Subcommittee of the American Academy of Neurology. Neurology. 2005;64:2008–20.
11. Zappia M, Albanese A, Bruno E, et al. Treatment of essential tremor: a systematic review of evidence and recommendations from the Italian Movement Disorders Association. J Neurol. 2013;260:714–40.
12. Diaz NL, Louis ED. Survey of medication usage patterns among essential tremor patients: movement disorder specialists vs. general neurologists. Parkinsonism Relat Disord. 2010;16:604–7.
13. Winkler GF, Young RR. The control of essential tremor by propranolol. Trans Am Neurol Assoc. 1971;96:66–8.
14. Larsen TA, Teravainen H. Beta 1 versus nonselective blockade in therapy of essential tremor. Adv Neurol. 1983;37:247–51.

15. Leigh PN, Jefferson D, Twomey A, Marsden CD. Beta-adrenoreceptor mechanisms in essential tremor; a double-blind placebo controlled trial of metoprolol, sotalol and atenolol. J Neurol Neurosurg Psychiatry. 1983;46:710–5.

16. Cleeves L, Findley LJ. Propranolol and propranolol-LA in essential tremor: a double blind comparative study. J Neurol Neurosurg Psychiatry. 1988;51:379–84.

17. Koller WC. Long-acting propranolol in essential tremor. Neurology. 1985;35:108–10.

18. Koller WC, Royse VL. Efficacy of primidone in essential tremor. Neurology. 1986;36:121–4.

19. Connor GS, Edwards K, Tarsy D. Topiramate in essential tremor: findings from double-blind, placebo-controlled, crossover trials. Clin Neuropharmacol. 2008;31:97–103.

20. Gironell A, Kulisevsky J, Barbanoj M, Lopez-Villegas D, Hernandez G, Pascual-Sedano B. A randomized placebo-controlled comparative trial of gabapentin and propranolol in essential tremor. Arch Neurol. 1999;56:475–80.

21. Ondo W, Hunter C, Vuong KD, Schwartz K, Jankovic J. Gabapentin for essential tremor: a multiple-dose, double-blind, placebo-controlled trial. Mov Disord. 2000;15:678–82.

22. Pahwa R, Lyons K, Hubble JP, et al. Double-blind controlled trial of gabapentin in essential tremor. Mov Disord. 1998;13:465–7.

23. Jefferson D, Jenner P, Marsden CD. Beta-adrenoreceptor antagonists in essential tremor. J Neurol Neurosurg Psychiatry. 1979;42:904–9.

24. Koller WC. Nadolol in essential tremor. Neurology. 1983;33:1076–7.

25. Huber SJ, Paulson GW. Efficacy of alprazolam for essential tremor. Neurology. 1988;38:241–3.

26. Gunal DI, Afsar N, Bekiroglu N, Aktan S. New alternative agents in essential tremor therapy: double-blind placebo-controlled study of alprazolam and acetazolamide. Neurol Sci. 2000;21:315–7.

27. Biary N, Koller W. Kinetic predominant essential tremor: successful treatment with clonazepam. Neurology. 1987;37:471–4.

28. Biary N, Bahou Y, Sofi MA, Thomas W, al Deeb SM. The effect of nimodipine on essential tremor. Neurology. 1995;45:1523–5.

29. Brin MF, Lyons KE, Doucette J, et al. A randomized, double masked, controlled trial of botulinum toxin type A in essential hand tremor. Neurology. 2001;56:1523–8.

30. Jankovic J, Schwartz K, Clemence W, Aswad A, Mordaunt J. A randomized, double-blind, placebo-controlled study to evaluate botulinum toxin type A in essential hand tremor. Mov Disord. 1996;11:250–6.
31. Pahwa R, Busenbark K, Swanson-Hyland EF, et al. Botulinum toxin treatment of essential head tremor. Neurology. 1995;45:822–4.
32. Hertegard S, Granqvist S, Lindestad PA. Botulinum toxin injections for essential voice tremor. Ann Otol Rhinol Laryngol. 2000;109:204–9.
33. Warrick P, Dromey C, Irish JC, Durkin L, Pakiam A, Lang A. Botulinum toxin for essential tremor of the voice with multiple anatomical sites of tremor: a crossover design study of unilateral versus bilateral injection. Laryngoscope. 2000;110:1366–74.
34. Pahwa R, Lyons KE, Wilkinson SB, et al. Comparison of thalamotomy to deep brain stimulation of the thalamus in essential tremor. Mov Disord. 2001;16:140–3.
35. Schuurman PR, Bosch DA, Bossuyt PM, et al. A comparison of continuous thalamic stimulation and thalamotomy for suppression of severe tremor. N Engl J Med. 2000;342:461–8.
36. Won E, Ellamushi HE, Samadani U, Baltuch GH. Essential tremor: patient selection, technique, and surgical results. In: Baltuch GH, Stern MB, editors. Surgical management of movement disorders. Boca Raton: Taylor & Francis Group; 2005. p. 111–21.
37. Gross RE, Krack P, Rodriguez-Oroz MC, Rezai AR, Benabid AL. Electrophysiological mapping for the implantation of deep brain stimulators for Parkinson's disease and tremor. Mov Disord. 2006;21 Suppl 14:S259–83.
38. Koller WC, Lyons KE, Wilkinson SB, Troster AI, Pahwa R. Long-term safety and efficacy of unilateral deep brain stimulation of the thalamus in essential tremor. Mov Disord. 2001;16:464–8.
39. Ondo W, Jankovic J, Schwartz K, Almaguer M, Simpson RK. Unilateral thalamic deep brain stimulation for refractory essential tremor and Parkinson's disease tremor. Neurology. 1998;51:1063–9.
40. Rehncrona S, Johnels B, Widner H, Tornqvist AL, Hariz M, Sydow O. Long-term efficacy of thalamic deep brain stimulation for tremor: double-blind assessments. Mov Disord. 2003;18:163–70.
41. Diamond A, Jankovic J. The effect of deep brain stimulation on quality of life in movement disorders. J Neurol Neurosurg Psychiatry. 2005;76:1188–93.

42. Hariz GM, Blomstedt P, Koskinen LO. Long-term effect of deep brain stimulation for essential tremor on activities of daily living and health-related quality of life. Acta Neurol Scand. 2008;118:387–94.

43. Carpenter MA, Pahwa R, Miyawaki KL, Wilkinson SB, Searl JP, Koller WC. Reduction in voice tremor under thalamic stimulation. Neurology. 1998;50:796–8.

44. Obwegeser AA, Uitti RJ, Turk MF, Strongosky AJ, Wharen RE. Thalamic stimulation for the treatment of midline tremors in essential tremor patients. Neurology. 2000;54:2342–4.

45. Binder DK, Rau GM, Starr PA. Risk factors for hemorrhage during microelectrode-guided deep brain stimulator implantation for movement disorders. Neurosurgery. 2005;56:722–32; discussion 722–732.

46. Baizabal Carvallo JF, Simpson R, Jankovic J. Diagnosis and treatment of complications related to deep brain stimulation hardware. Mov Disord. 2011;26:1398–406.

47. Obwegeser AA, Uitti RJ, Witte RJ, Lucas JA, Turk MF, Wharen Jr RE. Quantitative and qualitative outcome measures after thalamic deep brain stimulation to treat disabling tremors. Neurosurgery. 2001;48:274–81; discussion 281–274.

48. Anderson WS, Lenz FA. Surgery insight: deep brain stimulation for movement disorders. Nat Clin Pract Neurol. 2006;2:310–20.

49. Kondziolka D, Ong JG, Lee JY, Moore RY, Flickinger JC, Lunsford LD. Gamma knife thalamotomy for essential tremor. J Neurosurg. 2008;108:111–7.

50. Niranjan A, Jawahar A, Kondziolka D, Lunsford LD. A comparison of surgical approaches for the management of tremor: radiofrequency thalamotomy, gamma knife thalamotomy and thalamic stimulation. Stereotact Funct Neurosurg. 1999;72:178–84.

51. Elias WJ, Huss D, Voss T, et al. A pilot study of focused ultrasound thalamotomy for essential tremor. N Engl J Med. 2013;369:640–8.

52. Jankovic J, Cardoso F, Grossman RG, Hamilton WJ. Outcome after stereotactic thalamotomy for parkinsonian, essential, and other types of tremor. Neurosurgery. 1995;37:680–6; discussion 686–687.

53. Mohadjer M, Goerke H, Milios E, Etou A, Mundinger F. Long-term results of stereotaxy in the treatment of essential tremor. Stereotact Funct Neurosurg. 1990;54–55:125–9.

54. Nagaseki Y, Shibazaki T, Hirai T, et al. Long-term follow-up results of selective VIM-thalamotomy. J Neurosurg. 1986;65:296–302.
55. Niranjan A, Kondziolka D, Baser S, Heyman R, Lunsford LD. Functional outcomes after gamma knife thalamotomy for essential tremor and MS-related tremor. Neurology. 2000;55:443–6.
56. Siderowf A, Gollump SM, Stern MB, Baltuch GH, Riina HA. Emergence of complex, involuntary movements after gamma knife radiosurgery for essential tremor. Mov Disord. 2001;16:965–7.

Chapter 6
Case Studies

Case #1

Chief Complaint

Tremor of Hands.

History

This 18 year old right handed man initially noticed tremor of his right hand 3 months ago. Recently, he has noticed a slight tremor of his left hand as well. The tremor usually occurs only when he is holding objects such as a cup of coffee and during activity. There has been no change in his handwriting. He has no problem with eating, drinking from a glass full of liquids, or carrying out other activities of daily life. He has no history of thyroid disease. There is no history of antipsychotic/anti-emetic use or exposure to any toxins. He does not drink alcohol and denies using illicit drugs. Family history is notable for a father with a similar tremor, though more severe. He has no other medical problems.

A.Q. Rana, K.L. Chou, *Essential Tremor in Clinical Practice*, 63
In Clinical Practice, DOI 10.1007/978-3-319-14598-3_6,
© Springer International Publishing Switzerland 2015

Examination

He had mild amplitude, 9 Hz, flexion-extension tremors of both hands when outstretched, in wing beating position and on finger-nose-finger testing without any intention component. There was no resting tremor of the hands, bradykinesia or rigidity. There was no tremor of his voice, head, lips, chin, jaw, or lower extremities. The rest of the neurological examination, including tandem gait, was normal. His handwriting did not show any tremor. Spiral drawing showed a minimal tremor.

Diagnosis

Essential Tremor.

Case Discussion/Clinical Pearls

This patient presented with a 3 month history of bilateral action tremor of the hands, but no other complaints. While we do not know whether the tremors are responsive to alcohol, the presence of bilateral action tremors of the hands with a positive family history is highly suggestive of essential tremor.

While family history and alcohol responsiveness are supportive features of essential tremor, they do not have to be present to make the diagnosis. Enhanced physiologic tremor is in the differential diagnosis, but typically has a higher frequency. Nevertheless, thyroid studies should be done to rule out thyrotoxicosis. Because the patient is young, serum ceruloplasmin, 24 h urinary, and slit lamp examination for Kayser-Fleischer rings to rule out Wilson's disease may also be considered, though in this case, the presentation is fairly typical for essential tremor and it would be reasonable to defer testing until features that are atypical for essential tremor appear. The tremor is not interfering with activities of daily life at this point, so we would favour reassuring the patient that he does not have a neurodegenerative disorder such as Parkinson disease and monitor the condition. Treatment can be discussed when the tremors begin to interfere with activities.

Case #2

Chief Complaint

Tremor of both hands.

History

This is a 75 year old right handed man who noticed the gradual onset of bilateral hand tremor approximately 5 years ago. The tremors have worsened over that time, but particularly over the last 6 months. The tremor occurs when he is using his hands to perform activities, but he has also noticed them when his hands are in a resting position. His handwriting has become very coarse and tremulous over the last year. He finds difficulty drinking fluids, pouring, and using a spoon and fork while eating. He has stopped eating in public because of embarrassment. Others have mentioned that his head shakes, but he has not noticed it. Voice is normal. He is slightly slow in walking, a result that he attributes to arthritis; he may occasionally drool at night time while sleeping. His balance is not as great as it was before, and he may feel unsteady on his feet when he turns quickly. However, this has not resulted in any falls. He does not drink alcohol and there is no family history of tremor or Parkinson disease. He has no history of thyroid disease. There is no history of antipsychotic/antiemetic use or exposure to any toxins. Past medical history is significant only for hypertension, for which he takes an ACE inhibitor. He has no other medical problems and takes no other medications.

Examination

He had moderate amplitude, 8 Hz, flexion extension tremor of both hands when outstretched, in wing beating position and on finger-nose-finger testing without any intention component. There was mild amplitude, 8 Hz, flexion extension tremor of both hands with the hands resting in the lap, which disappeared on complete repose in supine position. There was a fine, high frequency, head shaking tremor, not worsened with different head positions. There was no tremor of head, voice, lips, chin, jaw or lower extremities. He had mild cogwheeling of both upper extremities at the elbows. There was no bradykinesia. His speed of walking was slightly slow, his gait was of an antalgic pattern. The rest of the neurological examination including tandem gait was normal. His handwriting and spiral drawing showed a moderate kinetic tremor.

Diagnosis

Essential tremor, interfering with activities of daily life.

Case Discussion/Clinical Pearls

This patient presents with bilateral tremor of the hands, present in a "rest" position, but worse with action, as well as a fine head tremor. Though his age and the presence of a rest tremor may bring up the possibility of Parkinson disease, this patient's tremor is worse with action, and when special attempts are made to completely relax the hands, the tremor disappears. The presence of a head tremor and a 5 year history without any evidence of bradykinesia on exam are other features of this case that are inconsistent with a diagnosis of Parkinson disease, making essential tremor the most likely diagnosis.

Thyroid studies would be reasonable tests to order if not done so already. No imaging tests are necessary. Because the tremors interfere with activities of daily living, the clinician should discuss treatment options with the patient. Both propranolol and primidone are acceptable first-line agents in this case. For propranolol, we recommend a starting dose of 20 mg three times daily or 60 mg daily in an extended release formulation. For primidone, we recommend starting with half of a 50 mg tablet at bedtime and titrating up on a weekly basis for effect.

Case #3

Chief Complaint

Tremor of both hands.

History

This 28 year old right handed Asian woman initially noticed tremor of both of her hands about 3 months ago. The tremor occurs mainly when holding objects and when using the hands. There is no tremor with the hands in a resting position. There is no significant change in handwriting. While there is tremor with drinking from a glass, eating, and putting on makeup, it is not so severe that she cannot perform them. She does not drink alcohol. Over the same time, she has noticed poor heat tolerance, increased perspiration, diarrhoea, occasional heart palpitations, and mild weight loss. There is no history of antipsychotic/antiemetic use or exposure to any toxins. She has no other medical problems. She is currently taking only a birth control pill.

Examination

She had a mild amplitude, 12 Hz, flexion extension tremor of both hands when outstretched. There was no tremor in the wing beating position or on the finger-nose-finger testing. Handwriting and spiral drawing did not reveal any tremor. There was no resting tremor in the hands and no tremor of voice, head, lips, chin, jaw, or lower extremities. The rest of the neurological examination, including tandem gait, was normal. Of note, her resting heart rate was 98.

Case Discussion/Clinical Pearls

This is a young woman with a mild action tremor of both hands. The main diagnostic considerations include enhanced physiologic tremor or essential tremor. Drug-induced tremor would also be a consideration if she was on a medication that could cause tremors. With her other constitutional symptoms, such as heat intolerance, palpitations and weight loss, thyroid studies were ordered. Her serum TSH was much below the normal range with an increase in the free T4 level. Thus, a diagnosis of tremor due to hyperthyroidism was made. She was referred for endocrinology consultation, and her tremors resolved once hyperthyroidism was under control.

Case #4

Chief Complaint

Head tremor.

History

This is a 47 year old right handed woman who initially noticed a head tremor 9 months ago. She reports that her head shakes side to side and tends to turn towards the left side. This is accompanied by soreness on the left side of her neck. By touching the side of her face she can bring her head back to a neutral position ceasing the tremor. However, as soon as she removes her hand, the head turns to the left and shakes again. The tremor is interfering with her social and household activities. There is no tremor involving her hands, voice, lips, jaw, chin or legs. She denies any change in her handwriting. She does not drink alcohol and there is no family history of tremor or other movement disorders. There is no history of antipsychotic/antiemetic use or exposure to any toxins. She has no known history of thyroid disease. Past medical history is significant for hypertension only for which she takes atenolol, a beta-blocker.

Examination

She had a mild amplitude, 5 Hz, side to side ("no-no") tremor of her head, though the tremor was jerky in nature. There was a 20–30° turn of her head towards the left side, and she had mildly decreased range of motion of her neck to the right side. The head tremor improved when turning to the left and worsened when turning to the right. There was no shift of her head. The right sternocleidomastoid muscle was mildly hypertrophied when compared to the left side. She was able to bring her head to a neutral position solely by touching the side of her head. Her left shoulder was higher and slightly anteriorly displaced, and palpation of the left side of her neck elicited a complaint of soreness. There was no tremor of her hands or upper extremities. There was no tremor of voice, lips, chin, jaw or lower extremities. The rest of the neurological examination, including tandem gait, was normal. Her handwriting and spiral drawing did not reveal any tremor.

Case Discussion/Clinical Pearls

The presence of a head tremor narrows the differential diagnosis considerably. The presence of dystonia on examination (turn of the head to the left with left shoulder elevation), the jerky nature of the tremor, and the presence of a sensory trick (tremor and head deviation are lessened when touching the cheek) is highly suggestive of a dystonic head tremor secondary to cervical dystonia.

The head tremor in essential tremor is almost always accompanied by bilateral hand tremors. Besides, the diagnosis of essential tremor cannot be made in the presence of dystonia. In a case such as this, it is important to ask about and closely review the medication log to make sure the patient has never been exposed to antipsychotic or antiemetic medications. The first line treatment for cervical dystonia is botulinum toxin. Oral medications are typically unhelpful in this condition.

Case #5

Chief Complaint

Essential tremor unresponsive to medications.

History

This is a 61 year old right handed man with a diagnosis of essential tremor. Tremors of the hands were first noticed over 20 years ago and have gradually worsened over time. Both hands are involved but it is worse on the left. He denies head, voice, chin, jaw or leg tremors. He has difficulty with many activities of daily living, including brushing his teeth, shaving, eating, and drinking. He has to be very careful eating soup, and needs to use two hands when drinking from a cup. His handwriting has become very illegible. Alcohol improves his tremor and he frequently has a glass of wine at social occasions so that others will not notice his tremor. There is no family history of tremor. There is no history of antipsychotic/antiemetic use or exposure to any toxins, nor is there a known history of thyroid disease. Past medical history is significant for hypertension, hypercholesterolemia, coronary artery disease, peripheral vascular disease, peripheral neuropathy, history of carotid stenosis status post right carotid endarter-ectomy, and low back pain. He is currently on primidone 300 mg daily and gabapentin 800 mg three times daily, but they do not help his tremor (though his gabapentin is more for his neuropathy). Other medications include a full aspirin daily, metoprolol 50 mg twice daily, losartan, amlodipine, and atorvastatin.

Examination

He had a moderate to severe amplitude, 8 Hz, flexion exten-sion tremor of both hands when outstretched, in a wing beat-ing position and on finger-nose-finger testing without any intention component. Tremor was slightly worse on the right than the left. There was no resting tremor. There was no tremor of his voice, head, lips, chin, jaw, or lower extremities. His handwriting and spiral drawing showed a moderate tremor. There was no evidence of bradykinesia or rigidity on examination. The rest of the neurological examination, including tandem gait, was normal.

Case Discussion/Clinical Pearls

The diagnosis is essential tremor. He has a long history of action tremors in the hands and his tremor is alcohol respon-sive. There is nothing in the history to suggest a drug-induced tremor or parkinsonism. His tremors are severe enough to interfere significantly with his day to day activities, and the patient is looking for other options.

He is currently on a high dose of primidone (300 mg daily) and gabapentin (2,400 mg daily), which have not been benefi-cial. Notes from this patient's treating physician state that he has failed all first-line agents for essential tremor, including a beta-blocker (metoprolol). However, not all beta-blockers are equally efficacious for essential tremor. Metoprolol is predominantly a central acting beta-blocker and is not as effective as propranolol, which acts more predominantly on peripheral beta receptors. Thus, there is one first-line agent for essential tremor that has not been tried: propranolol.

In this patient's case, a discussion was started with his cardiologist about possibly switching his beta-blocker from metoprolol to propranolol. However, because of the severity of the patient's cardiac disease, the cardiologist was reluctant to take him off the metoprolol. As a result, topiramate, was started and slowly titrated up to 100 mg twice daily. On this dose, he did not have any side effects, and his tremors were improved to the point where he was satisfied with the tremor control.

Case #6

Chief Complaint

Essential tremor unresponsive to medications.

History

This is a 65 year old right handed woman who initially noticed tremor in her hands when she was 11 years old. Initially, the tremor was exclusively in the hands but as she got older, she developed a head tremor as well. The hand tremors are noticeable only when she uses her hands and they interfere with her eating and drinking. She is unable to drink from a regular cup without spilling and needs to use a straw. She feels embarrassed eating in public because she spills food all over the place. She has also noticed deterioration of her handwriting, to the point where she can no longer sign for checks. There is a family history of similar tremor in her father and paternal grandfather. The tremors improve significantly after drinking a glass of wine. There is no history of antipsychotic/antiemetic use or exposure to any toxins, nor is there a known history of thyroid disease.

She currently takes propranolol 80 mg daily. While this helps her tremor somewhat, she is still significantly limited in her activities and her family practitioner will not increase the dose because of a heart rate consistently in the low 50s. Past treatments for tremor include primidone (which caused excessive sleepiness at a low dose even after continuing with the medication for 4 weeks), topiramate (which improved her tremor, but caused significant weight loss with no change in the appetite), gabapentin (which was ineffective and caused sleepiness) and atenolol (ineffective and caused her heart rate to go down to the 40s). Past medical history is significant only for irritable bowel symptoms and osteoporosis. Current medications include fexofenadine, vitamin D and hyoscyamine in addition to the propranolol.

Examination

She had a severe amplitude, 7–8 Hz, flexion extension tremor of the right hand and a moderate amplitude tremor of the left hand with both hands held outstretched, in a wing beating position and on finger-nose-finger testing without any intention component. There was no resting tremor. There was mild tremor of the voice with sustained phonation and a mild no-no tremor of the head. There was no tremor of the lips, chin, jaw, or lower extremities. When trying to sign her name, she could barely keep the pen on the paper. There was no rigidity in the arms on examination. Fine finger movements were slowed, likely because of tremor, and did not show decreased in amplitude with continued movements. The rest of the neurological examination, including tandem gait, was normal.

Case Discussion/Clinical Pearls

The diagnosis in this case is essential tremor. It has been present for a long time and has gradually worsened. The diagnosis is supported by a strong family history and alcohol responsiveness. There is nothing in the history to suggest a drug-induced tremor or parkinsonism. Her tremors are severe and greatly decrease her quality of life. She has been tried on the 2 first-line agents (primidone and propranolol) and 3 second-line agents (topiramate, gabapentin and atenolol) for essential tremor, and has had side effects or has been tried on adequate doses without tremor benefit. She is a good candidate for deep brain stimulation (DBS) therapy.

She underwent a comprehensive evaluation for DBS at a tertiary care center. A DBS electrode was implanted in the left VIM nucleus of the thalamus to help her right hand tremor. After a number of programming sessions to adjust the stimulator, her right hand tremor was well controlled and she was able to eat, drink, and write again without significant difficulty. Although she still had tremor in her left hand, it did not bother her enough to consider having a DBS electrode placed in her right thalamus.

Case #7

Chief Complaint

Hand tremor.

History

This 64 year old right handed man patient initially noticed an intermittent tremor of his right hand about 6 months ago, but the tremor has become more constant. The tremor is present only when his hand is at rest. It disappears when he uses his hand. He has not noticed tremor in the left hand. He has noticed that his handwriting has become small, but has no difficulty drinking from a glass or eating. There is some loss of dexterity in the right hand and he reports more difficulty cutting meat than before. He drinks a glass of wine each night, but has not noticed any improvement in his tremor.

There is no history of antipsychotic/antiemetic use or exposure to any toxins, nor is there a known history of thyroid disease. Past medical history is significant only for hypertension, and he only takes a baby aspirin and ramipril. Family history is significant for a mother with Parkinson disease and he is worried about this possibility.

Examination

He had a mild amplitude, 4 Hz, constant, pronation-supination rest tremor of the right hand, but no tremor when his hands were outstretched, in the wing beating position or on the finger-nose-finger testing. There was no tremor in the left hand. There was no tremor of voice, head, lips, chin, jaw, or lower extremities. There was rigidity noticeable at the right wrist, but nowhere else. There did not seem to be a particularly masked facial expression. His gait was normal, except that his tremor got worse when he was walking and there was a slight decrease in arm swing on the right compared to the left. Posture was normal.

Case Discussion/Clinical Pearls

This patient has a unilateral rest tremor, accompanied by rigidity. The presence of a rest tremor typically implies parkinsonism. This type of presentation is suggestive of Parkinson disease, and a good sustained response to levodopa would strongly support the diagnosis. Atypical forms of parkinsonism are in the differential, but would not be seriously considered unless the patient fails a trial of high dose levodopa. A dopamine transporter imaging study (DaTscan) could be considered, but this type of study can only distinguish essential tremor from parkinsonism, and the clinical course and examination are already inconsistent with a diagnosis of essential tremor.

While Parkinson disease is characterized by rest tremor, rigidity, bradykinesia and gait difficulties, not all four have to be present in order to make the diagnosis. In fact, if gait difficulty and falls are prominent at presentation of parkinsonism, an atypical form of parkinsonism should be considered. At initial presentation, bradykinesia and rigidity may be very subtle. The possible diagnosis of Parkinson disease was discussed with the patient. Treatment options, including side effects, were also discussed. Because none of his symptoms significantly interfered with his activities, he opted not to start treatment at this time.

Case #8

Chief Complaint

Hand tremor.

History

This 38 year old right handed man initially noticed tremor of both of his hands about 1½ years ago. The tremor occurs mainly when holding objects and during activity. He has noticed no tremor when his hands are in the resting position. His handwriting has become very coarse and shaky. In addition to difficulty with writing, he has difficulty drinking from a glass, eating, and carrying out other activities of daily life such as shaving and dressing. He does not drink alcohol. He has no history of thyroid disease. Past medical history is significant for a diagnosis of bipolar disorder, which has been stable on valproic acid (750 mg daily) for the last 2 years. He has no history of exposure to any toxins. The rest of the neurological inquiry was unremarkable.

Examination

He had a moderate amplitude, 8 Hz, flexion extension tremor of both hands with hands held outstretched, in the wing beating position, and on finger-nose-finger testing without any intention component. There was a very mild amplitude, 8 Hz, flexion extension tremor of both hands in the resting position. There was no tremor of his voice, head, lips, chin, jaw, or lower extremities. There was no rigidity or bradykinesia. His handwriting and spiral drawing showed moderate tremor. There was no micrographia on handwriting. The rest of the neurological examination, including tandem gait, was normal.

Case Discussion/Clinical Pearls

This patient has action tremor greater than resting tremor of both upper extremities in the absence of bradykinesia, rigidity or other parkinsonian signs. The examination could be consistent with a diagnosis of essential tremor, but the patient is on a medication, valproic acid, that can cause tremors. Thus, a diagnosis of drug-induced tremor was made.

The tremor is interfering with his daily activities. While medications such as propranolol and primidone can be used in drug-induced tremor, the best treatment would be to stop the inciting agent. Suggestions were made to his psychiatrist to change valproic acid to another mood stabilizer which would not exacerbate the tremor. (Please note that lithium is another mood stabilizing agent that is highly likely to cause tremor.)

Case #9

Chief Complaint

Hand tremor.

History

This 41 year old right handed man initially noticed tremor of both of his hands about 1 year ago. There has been no worsening of his tremor over time. The tremor is present in both of his hands while in the resting position, holding objects and during activity, much worse in the right hand than the left hand. His handwriting has become small and tremulous. He also has difficulty drinking from a glass and eating. He has also noticed slowness of movement and more of a shuffling gait over this period. He does not drink alcohol. He has no history of thyroid disease. Past medical history is significant for psychotic depression, but has been stable on sertraline (150 mg daily) and risperidone (2 mg twice daily) for the last 1½ years. There is a family history of depression, but not essential tremor or Parkinson disease.

Examination

He had a moderate amplitude, 8 HZ, flexion extension tremor of both hands in the resting position, while outstretched, in the wing beating position and on finger-nose-finger testing without any intention component. The tremor was worse on the right than the left. There was no tremor of voice, or lower extremities, but he did have an intermittent chin tremor. He had mild cogwheel rigidity of both upper extremities. There was mild bradykinesia with fine finger movements. Gait was slow with decreased stride length and decreased arm swing bilaterally. His handwriting was small and spiral drawing showed significant tremor. The rest of the neurological examination was normal.

Case Discussion/Clinical Pearls

This patient has an action and rest tremor of both upper extremities, accompanied by parkinsonian symptoms. The differential diagnosis of parkinsonism includes Parkinson disease, atypical parkinsonism and drug-induced parkinsonism. This patient has been on a medication, risperidone, which has dopamine blocking properties, so the likely diagnosis is drug-induced parkinsonism.

The symptoms, especially tremor, are interfering with his daily activities. The best treatment in this case is to remove the inciting agent. Suggestions were made to his psychiatrist to change risperidone to another agent with a better side effect profile. Among the atypical antipsychotics, only quetiapine and clozapine do not significantly worsen parkinsonism. Furthermore, it may take several months for symptoms of drug-induced parkinsonism to improve once the inciting agent is discontinued. In this case, risperidone was changed to quetiapine by his psychiatrist. He was seen 6 months later and his symptoms had significantly improved.

Case #10

Chief Complaint

Hand tremor.

History of Present Illness

This 25 year old left handed woman noticed left hand tremor a year ago, the day after a party at a friend's house. She remembers the exact day because she had food poisoning with nausea and vomiting, and as soon as her vomiting resolved, the tremor started. It was present both with action and at rest, though worse with action. About a month ago, the tremor spread to her right hand. The tremors are intermittent, and alternate between the left and right hand. When present, the tremor can last for hours, and it interferes with activities of daily life such as eating and drinking. In between episodes of tremor she feels normal. There has been no rigidity, bradykinesia, or gait difficulty. She does not drink alcohol. She has no history of thyroid disease. There is no history of antipsychotic/antiemetic use or exposure to any toxins, nor is there a known history of thyroid disease. There is no family history of tremor. Past medical history is significant only for an ovarian cyst and dysmenorrhea. Her only medications are iron pills.

Examination

She had an intermittent, flexion extension tremor of the right hand of variable amplitude and frequency, with the hands held outstretched. In the wing beating position, the right hand tremor disappeared and left hand tremor appeared, which also had variable amplitude and frequency. The hand tremor disappeared when performing opening-closing movements of the contralateral hand. There was mild tremor on finger-nose-finger testing bilaterally. There was no resting tremor of the hands. There was no tremor of the voice, head, lips, chin, jaw, or lower extremities. There was no rigidity or bradykinesia. Handwriting was normal. The rest of the neurological examination, including tandem gait, was normal.

Case Discussion/Clinical Pearls

This patient had a rather sudden onset of tremor that is now episodic, alternates between hands, and is distractible on examination (disappears with movements of the contralateral hand). All of these features are highly suggestive of a psychogenic or functional tremor. Psychological or psychiatric disturbances do not need to be present for the diagnosis to be made.

This diagnosis can be a difficult one for patients to accept, but the most important element in treatment is to convey the diagnosis to the patient. This should be done in a non-judgmental and empathetic, yet firm manner. Leaving doubt as to the diagnosis will only lead the patient to seek further consultations and testing. Non-pharmacologic approaches, including cognitive behavioural therapy and physical therapy may be helpful. If depression and anxiety are present, referral to a psychiatrist may also be helpful.

Appendices

Appendix A: Essential Tremor: A Short History

Numerous descriptions of tremor have been found in the ancient literature. In this chapter, we outline these descriptions which date from before the common era, to the early twentieth century, when the term "essential tremor" first started to appear in the medical literature.

- "Charaka Samhita", an ancient Indian text on internal medicine, dates back to around 300 B.C. It was written in Sanskrit language and is found at the University of Benares, India. In chapter 20, entitled Vepathu, a comprehensive description of tremors is documented [1, 2].
- In the second century, Greek physician Claudius Galen (130–201 AD) wrote "De Tremore", a short text on tremor and convulsions. In it, he distinguished between different types of tremors based on their causes and features. He thought that tremors were caused by a partial loss of force that moves the body. Heavy objects, fear, age, and sickness could cause this loss of force and result in tremors. Galen defined tremor as *"an involuntary alternating up-and-down motion of the limbs"*, and thought it could only be present with movement, not at rest [3]. He used the term *"palpitations"* to describe rest tremor.

A.Q. Rana, K.L. Chou, *Essential Tremor in Clinical Practice*,   81
In Clinical Practice, DOI 10.1007/978-3-319-14598-3,
© Springer International Publishing Switzerland 2015

- Ibn-Sina (Avicenna; 980–1036 AD), was an Arabic philosopher, physician and author and dubbed the "prince and chief of physicians" [4]. He wrote over 450 works, and his "Canon of Medicine" is one of the most influential textbooks on medicine. In it, he writes that tremor is "a kind of neurological disorder which is a combination of involuntary movement with voluntary movement or static state." [5]

- The following statement by Leonardo da Vinci (1452–1519) in his notebooks describes the tremor of the hand and head. He writes "*for you will see palsied and shivering persons move, and their trembling limbs, as their head and hands, quake without leave from their soul and their soul with all its power cannot prevent their members from trembling*" [6].

- Franciscus de le Boë (Sylvius: 1614–1672), a professor of medicine in Leiden in 1658, distinguishes between action tremor and rest tremor in his *Opera Medica*. He describes "*the tremulous motion…that stops when the body is at rest, and that is reinstated whenever the same movement is repeated*" and an "involuntary" or rest tremor [3].

- Gerard van Swieten (1700–1772) continued to write of the distinction between action and rest tremor, writing in his *Commentaries on the aphorisms of Boerhaave*, "Furthermore, two kinds of tremor are observed: one occurs while someone rests and lays in bed; this tremor is involuntary, and may alternately stop and soon reappear, so that a limb is set into motion; the patient cannot control this tremor, even if he wants to: the other tremor appears when the patient wants to move the whole body, or parts of it." [3]

- Francois Boissier de Sauvages de Lacroix (1706–1767) was a French physician who established a methodical nosology for diseases. In his writings, he also distinguished action tremor from rest tremor "by observing, that [in rest tremor] the tremulous parts leap, and as it were vibrate, even when supported: whilst every other tremor, he observes, ceases, when the voluntary exertion for moving the limb stops, or the part is supported, but returns when we will the limb to move." [7]

- James Parkinson (1755–1824) was a general practitioner in London, England who in 1817 published an essay on "Shaking Palsy" in which he described six individuals affected with the condition that now bears his name [7]. He described this condition as having "*Involuntary tremulous motion, with lessened muscular power, in parts not in action and even when supported, with a propensity to bend the trunk forwards, and to pass from a walking to a running pace, the senses and intellect being uninjured.*" However, later in his essay, he distinguishes the rest tremor seen in Parkinson disease from the action tremor that we associate with essential tremor, and cites de le Boë Sylvius and Sauvages as previous physicians who pointed out this important difference.

- In 1836, G.F. Most was the first to report several cases of tremor in a single family [8].

- American neurologist Charles Dana (1852–1935) is credited with the first description of hereditary essential tremor in 1887 [8, 9]. Dana described a postural tremor that occurred in several New York families. He characterized the different body parts which were affected with tremor, severity of tremor, age of onset, absence of tremor during sleep and no effect of tremor on mortality. Dana thought essential tremor was related to neurosis, epilepsy, high intellect and psychosis. However, he described that the condition increased with alcohol [8, 9].

- In the 1870s–1890s, variants of the term essential tremor started to appear in the medical literature [10]. Pietro Burresi, a Professor of Medicine in Italy, used the term *tremor semplice essenziale* (simple essential tremor) in 1874. His case report was of a young man with action tremors of the hands and head tremor, but was not familial. In 1879, Edoardo Maragliano, another Italian, used the term *tremore essenziale congenito* (i.e., essential congenital tremor), because his case was of a man with action tremors of the hands from almost birth. Anton Nagy (1863–1935), in

Austria, reported a young woman with severe familial tremor in 1890. In this woman's family, 19 had tremor over 6 generations. He used the term *essentieller Tremor* (essential tremor). Finally, Fulgence Raymond (1842–1910) at the Salpe^trie`re Hospital in Paris reported "a variety of tremor that has hereditary component, which should be named *essential tremor*, because it occurs independently from any other symptom which would make us think of brain injury or intoxication." [10]

References

1. Dass RK. Charaka Samhita: a critical review. J Ayurveda Holist Med. 2013;1:20–2.
2. Ovallath S, Deepa P. The history of parkinsonism: descriptions in ancient Indian medical literature. Mov Disord Off J Mov Disord Soc. 2013;28:566–8.
3. Koehler PJ, Keyser A. Tremor in Latin texts of Dutch physicians: 16th–18th centuries. Mov Disord Off J Mov Disord Soc. 1997;12:798–806.
4. Namazi MR. Avicenna, 980–1037. Am J Psychiatry. 2001;158:1796.
5. Zargaran A, Zarshenas MM, Mehdizadeh A, Mohagheghzadeh A. Management of tremor in medieval Persia. J Hist Neurosci. 2013;22:53–61.
6. Richter JP. The notebooks of Leonardo da Vinci, vol 2; 1888. Available at http://www.gutenberg.org/ebooks/5000
7. Parkinson J. An essay on the Shaking Palsy. London: Sherwood, Neely, and Jones; 1817.
8. Dana CL. Hereditary tremor: a hitherto undescribed form of motor neurosis. Am J Med Sci. 1887;94:386–93.
9. Lanska DJ. Chapter 33: the history of movement disorders. Handb Clin Neurol. 2010;95:501–46.
10. Louis ED, Broussolle E, Goetz CG, Krack P, Kaufmann P, Mazzoni P. Historical underpinnings of the term essential tremor in the late 19th century. Neurol. 2008;71:856–59.

Appendix B: Resources for Essential Tremor

International Essential Tremor Foundation

A non-profit organization dedicated to providing educational information, services and support to those affected by essential tremor (ET), and to health care providers, while promoting and funding ET research.

IETF
P.O. Box 14005
Lenexa, KS 66285-4005
Toll-free Phone: 888.387.3667
E-mail: info@essentialtremor.org
http://www.essentialtremor.org/Contact-Us

Lift Labs

A company working to develop new technologies for people with Essential Tremor and Parkinson's Disease. Makers of the Liftware spoon.

Lift Labs
1777 Yosemite Ave, Suite 235
San Francisco, CA 94124
Phone: 415.894.LIFT
E-mail: info@liftlabsdesign.com
http://www.liftlabsdesign.com/

Medtronic, Inc.

A medical technology company that developed deep brain stimulation (DBS) therapy for movement disorders, including essential tremor. As of this printing, only Medtronic, Inc. offers FDA-approved DBS systems.

Medtronic, Inc.
710 Medtronic Parkway
Minneapolis, Minnesota
55432-5604
USA
Toll-free: (800) 633-8766
Worldwide: (763) 514-4000
http://www.medtronic.com

Tremor Action Network

A volunteer non-profit organization founded by people diagnosed with essential tremor, cervical dystonia (spasmodic torticollis), and tremor related neurological movement disorders to spread awareness of essential tremor and tremor related disorders by advocating for a cure through research.

Tremor Action Network
P.O. Box 5013
Pleasanton, CA 94566
Phone: (510) 681-6565
http://www.tremoraction.org

WE MOVE – Worldwide Education and Awareness for Movement Disorders

WE MOVE is a not-for-profit organization dedicated to educating and informing patients, professionals and the public about the latest clinical advances, management and treatment options for neurologic movement disorders.

WE MOVE
5731 Mosholu Avenue
Bronx, NY 10471
E-mail: wemove@wemove.org
http://www.wemove.org

Index

A.Q. Rana, K.L. Chou, *Essential Tremor in Clinical Practice*,   87
In Clinical Practice, DOI 10.1007/978-3-319-14598-3,
© Springer International Publishing Switzerland 2015